Pocket Guide to Practical Psychopharmacology

Andrea Fagiolini
Alessandro Cuomo
Roger S. McIntyre

Pocket Guide to Practical Psychopharmacology

SSRIs and SNRIs in Clinical Practice

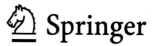 Springer

Andrea Fagiolini
Department of Molecular
Medicine
University of Siena
Siena, Siena, Italy

Alessandro Cuomo
Division of Psychiatry,
Department of Molecular
Medicine
University of Siena
Siena, Siena, Italy

Roger S. McIntyre
University Health Network
University of Toronto
Toronto, ON, Canada

ISBN 978-3-031-80489-2   ISBN 978-3-031-80490-8   (eBook)
https://doi.org/10.1007/978-3-031-80490-8

This Springer imprint is published by the registered company Springer Nature
Switzerland AG
The registered company address is: Gewerbestrasse 11, 6330 Cham, Switzerland

If disposing of this product, please recycle the paper.

Contents

Introduction

1

1.1 Choosing an Antidepressant

Depression is a complex and heterogeneous mental disorder characterized by a wide range of symptoms. These symptoms include, but are not limited to, persistent sadness, loss of interest or pleasure, changes in weight or appetite, insomnia or hypersomnia, psychomotor agitation or retardation, fatigue, feelings of worthlessness or guilt, diminished ability to think or concentrate, and recurrent thoughts of death or suicide. Effective treatment of depression often requires a personalized approach that takes into account the individual's specific symptom profile, the efficacy of different medications on these symptoms, and the pharmacodynamics of these medications [1, 2].

Therefore, the selection of an antidepressant requires consideration of several factors, including an individual's specific symptoms, medical history, the pharmacodynamic profile of the medication, potential side effects, and personal preferences. Below are some important criteria to consider when choosing an antidepressant:

1. Type of depression: Different antidepressants target specific neurotransmitters in the brain [3, 4]. For example, selective serotonin reuptake inhibitors (SSRIs) primarily affect serotonin levels, while serotonin–norepinephrine reuptake inhibi-

A. Fagiolini et al., *Pocket Guide to Practical Psychopharmacology*, https://doi.org/10.1007/978-3-031-80490-8_1

tors (SNRIs) affect both serotonin and norepinephrine. However, certain SSRIs may also affect norepinephrine levels (e.g., paroxetine, at higher doses) or dopamine levels (e.g., sertraline, at higher doses). Tricyclic antidepressants (TCAs) and monoamine oxidase inhibitors (MAOIs) are other classes that work in different ways.

2. Side effects: Antidepressants can have a variety of side effects, ranging from mild to severe [5]. Common side effects include sexual dysfunction, weight gain, dry mouth, dizziness, nausea, and difficulty sleeping. For example, patients whose depressive symptoms include loss of appetite may benefit from, rather than suffer from, an antidepressant that has increased appetite as a side effect. Conversely, patients who have already gained too much weight and are very concerned about weight gain may want a medication with the lowest possible risk of weight gain.

3. Medical history: Medical history, including pre-existing medical conditions, allergies, and current medications, should be considered when choosing an antidepressant [6]. Antidepressants may interact with other medications or worsen certain medical conditions.

4. Safety and tolerability: Some antidepressants have a better safety profile than others, such as the risk of overdose. MAOIs, for example, have strict dietary restrictions due to potentially dangerous interactions with certain foods and other medications. Individuals also vary in their ability to tolerate side effects, so it is important to find a medication that is well tolerated [7].

5. Response to previous treatments: People who have responded to (and tolerated) an antidepressant in the past may respond to the same medication when experiencing a new depressive episode. However, this is not true for everyone [8].

6. Lifestyle factors: Considerations such as dosing frequency, potential for weight gain, and effect on sexual function may influence the choice, especially if these factors are important in the patient's daily life.

7. Patient preferences: Personal preferences, including pill versus liquid preference, potential for once-daily dosing, or preference for a medication with a shorter half-life, should be considered.

1.2   Dosage and Administration

It is usually recommended to start an antidepressant at the lowest effective dose with the fewest side effects, in the most optimal balanced manner. If there is no improvement in 2–4 weeks, an increase in dose should be considered with appropriate monitoring of side effects. However, if a partial response is achieved after 1–2 weeks, maintaining the initial dosage could lead to remission during the following 8 weeks. The maximum recommended dose could be administered if the patient does not achieve remission and tolerates a higher drug dose.

1.3   Onset of Action

Improvement following the introduction of an antidepressant may be observed as early as 1 or 2 weeks after treatment is started. However, if the patient does not continue to improve, an increase in dose may be considered [9]. It is usually not recommended to switch to a new antidepressant before the maximum tolerated dose has been tried [10].

1.4   Duration of Treatment

Typically, treatment of a single depressive episode should continue for 1 year after improvement is achieved, while long-term maintenance dosing should be recommended for patients with recurrent depressive episodes [11].

1.5   Drug Interactions

Drug–drug interactions due to pharmacodynamic (additive, synergistic, or antagonistic effects) or pharmacokinetic (altered absorption, distribution, metabolism, or excretion) mechanisms between an antidepressant and another agent are possible [12]. Hepatic cytochrome CYP450 is often involved in the metabolism of antidepressants. Therefore, drugs with enhanced inhibitory or inducing CYP450 properties, either between two different antidepressants or between an antidepressant and another agent (i.e., anticonvulsant, antipsychotic, or opiate), should be considered very carefully [13].

1.6   Suicidality

Antidepressant treatment may be associated with an increased risk of suicidality, particularly in children and adolescents. Therefore, in 2004, the FDA placed a black box warning on all antidepressant packages for children, adolescents, and young adults up to 25 years of age [14]. In our experience, the risk is higher in the presence of symptoms such as psychomotor agitation, irritability, severe insomnia, active suicidality, and inner tension. In these cases, we usually do not start an antidepressant until the above symptoms have improved with a medication such as a benzodiazepine or quetiapine (which is approved for patients with major depressive disorder who do not respond to a classical antidepressant) or another medication (e.g., antimanic agents) that can treat these symptoms. Patients with suicidal ideation may be considered for lithium treatment and will usually be admitted for inpatient treatment unless they have a caregiver who can provide a level of safety similar to that of inpatient units.

1.7   Next Step Treatments

Patients who have not achieved remission after 4 or more weeks of depression treatment should be considered for adjunctive psychotherapy, augmentation strategy (i.e., lithium, esketamine, atypical antipsychotics), or switching to another class of antidepressant [14].

References

1. Taliaz D, Spinrad A, Barzilay R, Barnett-Itzhaki Z, Averbuch D, Teltsh O, Schurr R, Darki-Morag S, Lerer B. Optimizing prediction of response to antidepressant medications using machine learning and integrated genetic clinical and demographic data. Translational. Psychiatry. 2021;11(1) https://doi.org/10.1038/s41398-021-01488-3.

2. Maj M, Stein DJ, Parker G, Zimmerman M, Fava GA, De Hert M, Demyttenaere K, McIntyre RS, Widiger T, Wittchen H-U. The clinical characterization of the adult patient with depression aimed at personalization of management. World Psychiatry. 2020;19(3):269–93. https://doi.org/10.1002/wps.v19.3; https://doi.org/10.1002/wps.20771.

3. Jarończyk M, Walory J. Novel molecular targets of antidepressants. Molecules. 2022;27(2):533. https://doi.org/10.3390/molecules27020533.

4. Machado-Vieira R, Henter ID, Zarate CA Jr. New targets for rapid antidepressant action. Prog Neurobiol. 2017;152:21–37. https://doi.org/10.1016/j.pneurobio.2015.12.001.

5. Zhou Q, Li X, Yang D, Xiong C, Xiong Z. A comprehensive review and meta-analysis of neurological side effects related to second-generation antidepressants in individuals with major depressive disorder. Behav Brain Res. 2023;447:114431. https://doi.org/10.1016/j.bbr.2023.114431.

6. Runia N, Yücel DE, Lok A, de Jong K, Denys DAJP, van Wingen GA, Bergfeld IO. The neurobiology of treatment-resistant depression: a systematic review of neuroimaging studies. Neurosci Biobehav Rev. 2022;132:433–48. https://doi.org/10.1016/j.neubiorev.2021.12.008.

7. Nye A, Delgadillo J, Barkham M. Efficacy of personalized psychological interventions: a systematic review and meta-analysis. J Consult Clin Psychol. 2023;91(7):389–97. https://doi.org/10.1037/ccp0000820.

8. Simon GE, Perlis RH. Personalized medicine for depression: can we match patients with treatments? Am J Psychiatry. 2010;167(12):1445–55. https://doi.org/10.1176/appi.ajp.2010.09111680.

9. Kendrick T, Taylor D, Johnson CF. Which first-line antidepressant? Br J Gen Pract. 2019;69(680):114–5. https://doi.org/10.3399/bjgp19X701405.

10. Low Y, Setia S, Lima G. Drug-drug interactions involving antidepressants: focus on desvenlafaxine. Neuropsychiatr Dis Treat. 2018;14:567–80. Published 2018 Feb 19. https://doi.org/10.2147/NDT.S157708.

11. Chiew AL, Buckley NA. The serotonin toxidrome: shortfalls of current diagnostic criteria for related syndromes. Clin Toxicol (Phila). 2022;60(2):143–58. https://doi.org/10.1080/15563650.2021.1993242.

12. Hoffelt C, Gross T. A review of significant pharmacokinetic drug interactions with antidepressants and their management. Ment Health Clin. 2016;6(1):35–41. Published 2016 Mar 8. https://doi.org/10.9740/mhc.2016.01.035.

13. Cai H, Xie XM, Zhang Q, et al. Prevalence of suicidality in major depressive disorder: a systematic review and meta-analysis of comparative studies. Front Psychiatry. 2021;12:690130. Published 2021 Sep 16. https://doi.org/10.3389/fpsyt.2021.690130.

14. McIntyre RS, Alsuwaidan M, Baune BT, Berk M, Demyttenaere K, Goldberg JF, Gorwood P, Ho R, Kasper S, Kennedy SH, Ly-Uson J, Mansur RB, McAllister-Williams RH, Murrough JW, Nemeroff CB, Nierenberg AA, Rosenblat JD, Sanacora G, Schatzberg AF, Shelton R, Stahl SM, Trivedi MH, Vieta E, Vinberg M, Williams N, Young AH, Maj M. Treatment-resistant depression: definition, prevalence, detection, management, and investigational interventions. World Psychiatry. 2023 Oct;22(3):394–412. https://doi.org/10.1002/wps.21120. PMID: 37713549; PMCID: PMC10503923

SSRIs

2

2.1 Citalopram

2.1.1 Introduction and Indications

Citalopram (Fig. 2.1) is one of the first-line treatments for depression and anxiety disorders [1, 2].

Citalopram, an SSRI, was initially approved by the United States Food and Drug Administration in 1998. It is approved to treat major depressive disorders (MDD) in adults [2].

2.1.2 Structure of Citalopram (Fig. 2.1) [3]

2.1.3 What Are the Dosing Regimens for Citalopram?

Citalopram should be administered once daily with or without meals (Fig. 2.2).

© The Author(s), under exclusive license to Springer Nature
Switzerland AG 2024
A. Fagiolini et al., *Pocket Guide to Practical Psychopharmacology*,
https://doi.org/10.1007/978-3-031-80490-8_2

Fig. 2.1 Structure of citalopram

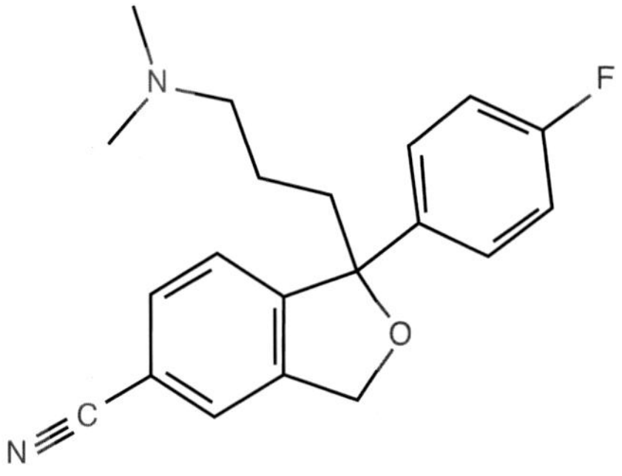

- **Initial dose:** 20 mg once a day.
- **After a week of dosing:** The dose may be increased to 40 mg once daily in patients younger than 60 years of age.
- **Elderly patients over 60 years of age, CYP2C19 poor metabolizers, and patients with hepatic impairment:** For these patients, the maximum recommended dose of citalopram is 20 mg once daily [2, 4].

2.1.4 What Are the Pharmacokinetic Profiles of Citalopram?

Absorption, Distribution, Metabolism, and Excretion of Citalopram [2] (**Fig. 2.3**).

2.1.5 What Are the Pharmacodynamic Profiles of Citalopram?

In vitro and in vivo animal studies indicated that citalopram has minimal effects on norepinephrine (NE) and dopamine (DA) neuronal reuptake.

Citalopram has little or no affinity for $5\text{-}HT_{1A}$, $5\text{-}HT_{2A}$, $\alpha_1\text{-}$, $\alpha_2\text{-}$, and β-adrenergic, dopamine D_1 and D_2, histamine H_1, muscarinic cholinergic, benzodiazepine, and gamma-aminobutyric acid receptors [2].

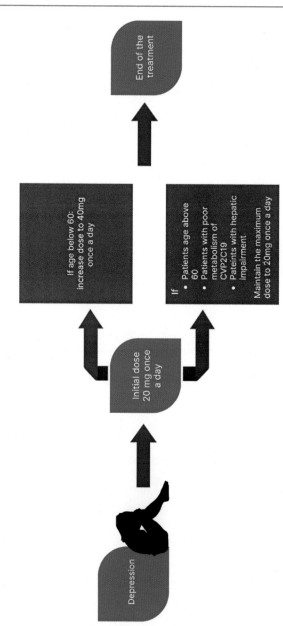

Fig. 2.2 Dosing regimens for citalopram

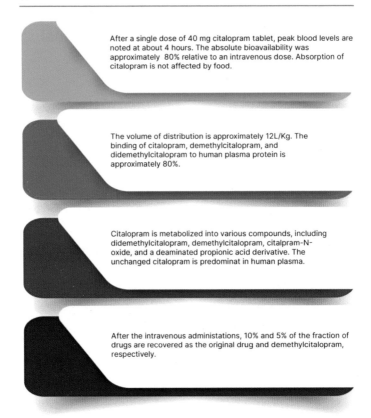

After a single dose of 40 mg citalopram tablet, peak blood levels are noted at about 4 hours. The absolute bioavailability was approximately 80% relative to an intravenous dose. Absorption of citalopram is not affected by food.

The volume of distribution is approximately 12L/Kg. The binding of citalopram, demethylcitalopram, and didemethylcitalopram to human plasma protein is approximately 80%.

Citalopram is metabolized into various compounds, including didemethylcitalopram, demethylcitalopram, citalpram-N-oxide, and a deaminated propionic acid derivative. The unchanged citalopram is predominat in human plasma.

After the intravenous administations, 10% and 5% of the fraction of drugs are recovered as the original drug and demethylcitalopram, respecively.

Fig. 2.3   Absorption, distribution, metabolism, and excretion of citalopram

2.1.6   What Is the Mechanism of Action of Citalopram?

Although the mechanism of action of citalopram is unclear, it could be related to serotonergic activity potentiation in the central nervous system (CNS) due to its inhibition of CNS neuronal reuptake of serotonin (Fig. 2.4) [2].

Fig. 2.4 Mechanism of action of citalopram

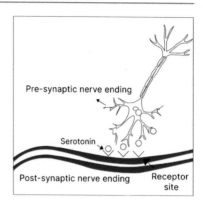

2.1.7 What Happens if Citalopram Is Discontinued?

Abrupt discontinuation is not recommended with citalopram, as abrupt cessation of these drugs is associated with a discontinuation syndrome (Fig. 2.5). Therefore, the discontinuation of these drugs should be accomplished with gradual dose tapering.

Adverse reactions after abrupt discontinuation of serotonergic antidepressants, such as citalopram, include nausea, dysphoric mood, anxiety, sweating, agitation, irritability, dizziness, headache, sensory disturbances, tremor, emotional lability, confusion, lethargy, insomnia, tinnitus, seizures, and hypomania [2].

2.1.8 What Are the Contraindications of Citalopram?

Contraindications of Citalopram (Fig. 2.6) [2].

2.1.9 What Are the Warnings and Precautions of Citalopram?

The warnings and precautions for patients using citalopram include the following (Fig. 2.7) [2]:

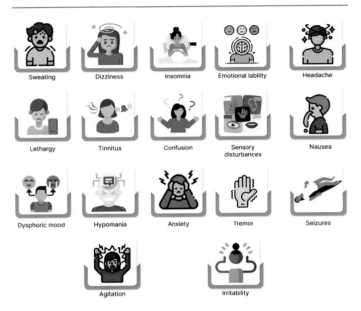

Fig. 2.5 Abrupt discontinuation of citalopram [2]

- **QT prolongation and torsade de pointes:** Dose-related QTc prolongation, ventricular tachycardia, torsade de pointes, and sudden death have been reported. Citalopram should be avoided in patients with bradycardia, hypokalemia, congenital long QT syndrome, hypomagnesemia, recent acute myocardial infarction, or decompensated heart failure and in those taking other medications that prolong the QTc interval. Citalopram should be discontinued in those with persistent QTc measurements >500 ms. Electrolyte levels should be monitored in those at high risk for hypomagnesemia or hypokalemia.
- **Serotonin syndrome:** The risk of serotonin syndrome increases when citalopram is used with other serotonergic agents. However, there is a risk even when taken alone. Citalopram should be discontinued and supportive measures initiated if serotonin syndrome occurs.
- **Increased risk of bleeding:** Concurrent use of other medications, including nonsteroidal anti-inflammatory drugs, aspirin, and other antiplatelet and anticoagulant medications, may increase the bleeding risk.

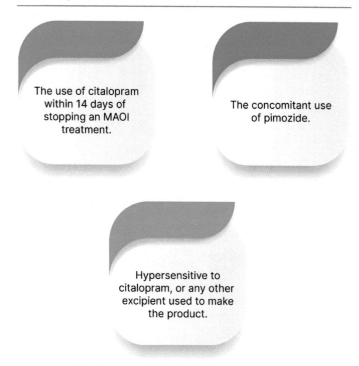

Fig. 2.6 Contraindications of citalopram. MAOI: Monoamine oxidase inhibitor

- **Activation of mania/hypomania:** Patients should be evaluated for bipolar disorder. In patients with bipolar disorder, the use of a concomitant mood stabilizer or other antimanic agent (e.g., an antipsychotic) should be considered.
- **Seizures:** Citalopram should be used cautiously in patients with a seizure disorder.
- **Angle-closure glaucoma:** Citalopram is not recommended in those with untreated anatomically narrow angle glaucoma.
- **Hyponatremia:** Hyponatremia and a syndrome of inappropriate antidiuretic hormone secretion are possible.
- **Sexual dysfunction:** Citalopram may lead to sexual dysfunction.

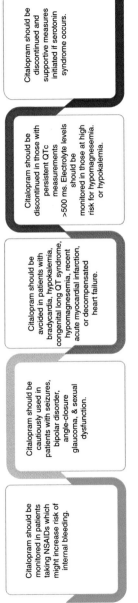

Fig. 2.7 Warnings and precautions for patients using citalopram

2.1.10 What Are the Most Common or Most Worrisome Adverse Reactions Associated with Citalopram?

The most common adverse reaction of citalopram is ejaculation disorder, i.e., primarily ejaculation delay [2, 4].

Adverse reactions associated with citalopram (Fig. 2.8) [2, 4].

2.1.11 What Are the Clinically Important Drug Interactions Associated with Citalopram?

Clinically Important Drug Interactions Associated with Citalopram (Table 2.1) [2].

2.1.12 Use in Special Populations (Fig. 2.9)?

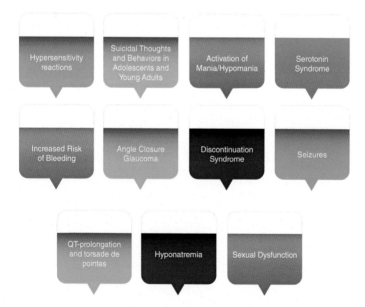

Fig. 2.8 Adverse reactions associated with citalopram

Table 2.1 Clinically important drug interactions associated with citalopram

Monoamine oxidase inhibitors (MAOIs)	Concomitant use of citalopram and MAOIs increases the risk of serotonin syndrome. Citalopram is contraindicated in those on MAOI therapy, such as intravenous methylene blue and linezolid
Drug that prolongs the QTC interval	Concomitant use of citalopram with these drugs can cause additional QT prolongation; thus, concomitant administration is contraindicated
Pimozide	Concomitant use of citalopram and pimozide increases the plasma concentration of pimozide; thus, concomitant administration of these two drugs is contraindicated
CYP2C19 inhibitors	Concomitant use of citalopram with these drugs increases the risk of ventricular arrhythmia and/or QT prolongation compared to using citalopram alone. The maximum recommended dose of citalopram is 20 mg when co-administered with a CYP2C19 inhibitor
Drugs that interfere with hemostasis	Concomitant use of these drugs with citalopram increases the risk of bleeding. Patients should be informed about this risk, and the international normalized ratio should be monitored
Serotonergic drugs	Concomitant use of serotonergic drugs and citalopram increases the risk of serotonin syndrome. The patient should be monitored during citalopram initiation and dose up-titration. Citalopram should be discontinued in case of serotonin syndrome

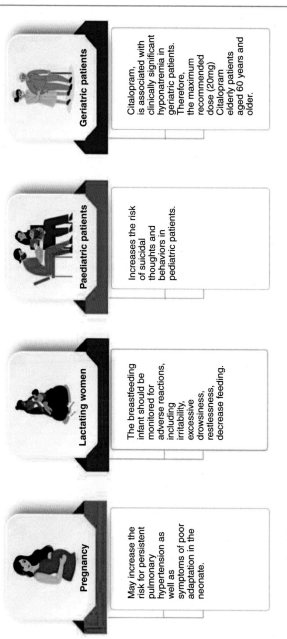

Geriatric patients

Citalopram, is associated with clinically significant hyponatremia in geriatric patients. Therefore, the maximum recommended dose (20mg) Citalopram elderly patients aged 60 years and older.

Paediatric patients

Increases the risk of suicidal thoughts and behaviors in pediatric patients.

Lactating women

The breastfeeding infant should be monitored for adverse reactions, including irritability, excessive drowsiness, restlessness, decrease feeding.

Pregnancy

May increase the risk for persistent pulmonary hypertension as well as symptoms of poor adaptation in the neonate.

Fig. 2.9 Citalopram in special populations

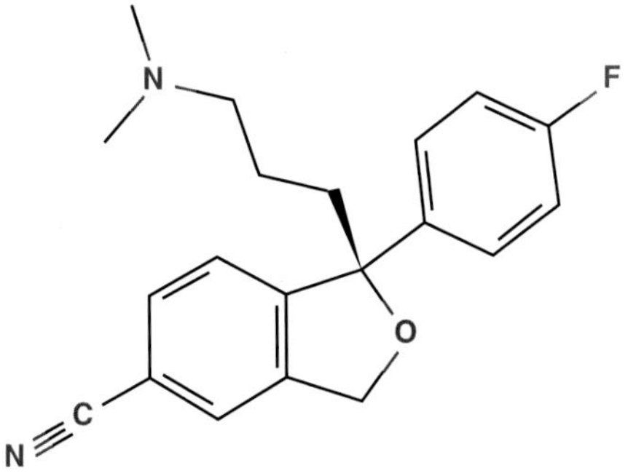

Fig. 2.10 Structure of escitalopram

2.2   Escitalopram

2.2.1   Introduction and Indications

Escitalopram, an SSRI and S-enantiomer of citalopram, was initially approved by the United States Food and Drug Administration in 2002. In the United States, it is indicated in the treatment of major depressive disorder (MDD) in adults and pediatric patients 12 years of age and older and in the treatment of generalized anxiety disorder (GAD) in adults and pediatric patients 7 years and older [5]. The indications may be different in other countries.

Structure of Escitalopram (Fig. 2.10) [6].

2.2.2   What Are the Dosing Regimens for Escitalopram (Fig. 2.11)?

Escitalopram should be administered once daily with or without food; it can be administered in the morning or evening. The dose of escitalopram should be reduced gradually while discontinuing the treatment [5].

Dosing Regimen of Escitalopram in Patients with Renal and/ or Hepatic Impairment (Fig. 2.12) [5].

What Are the Dosing Regimens for Escitalopram (Table 2.2)?

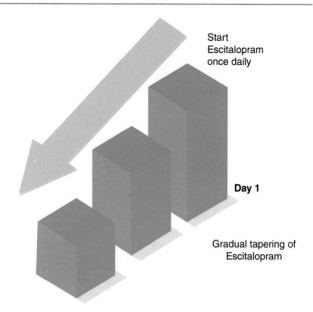

Fig. 2.11 Dosing regimens for escitalopram

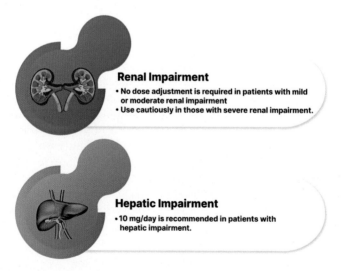

Fig. 2.12 Dosing regimen of escitalopram in patients with renal and/or hepatic impairment

Table 2.2   Dosing regimens for escitalopram

Indication	Starting daily dose	Recommended dose	Maximum daily dose
Major depression in adults	10 mg	10 mg	20 mg
Major depression in pediatric patients 12 years and older	10 mg	10 mg	20 mg
Generalized anxiety disorder in adults	10 mg	10 mg	20 mg
Generalized anxiety disorder in pediatric patients 7 years and older	10 mg	10 mg	20 mg

2.2.3   What Are the Pharmacokinetic Profiles of Escitalopram?

Among the SSRIs, escitalopram is one of the drugs that may be the best tolerated with the least chances of having serious pharmacokinetic interactions [4].

Absorption, Distribution, Metabolism, and Excretion of Escitalopram (Fig. 2.13) [5].

2.2.4   What Are the Pharmacodynamic Profiles of Escitalopram?

In vitro and in vivo animal studies indicated that escitalopram, an SSRI, has minimal effects on dopamine and norepinephrine neuronal reuptake. It is $\geq$100-fold more potent than citalopram in inhibiting 5-HT reuptake and 5-HT neuronal firing rate. Escitalopram has no or minimal affinity for serotonergic (5-HT_{1-7}) or other receptors, such as α- and β-adrenergic, benzodiazepine receptors, histamine (H_{1-3}), muscarinic (M_{1-5}), and dopamine (D_{1-5}). Escitalopram does not bind to or has little affinity for various ion channels, such as Na^+, Cl^-, K^+, and Ca^{++} channels [5].

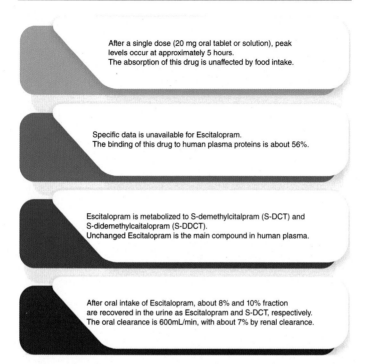

After a single dose (20 mg oral tablet or solution), peak levels occur at approximately 5 hours.
The absorption of this drug is unaffected by food intake.

Specific data is unavailable for Escitalopram.
The binding of this drug to human plasma proteins is about 56%.

Escitalopram is metabolized to S-demethylcitalpram (S-DCT) and S-didemethylcaitalopram (S-DDCT).
Unchanged Escitalopram is the main compound in human plasma.

After oral intake of Escitalopram, about 8% and 10% fraction are recovered in the urine as Escitalopram and S-DCT, respectively.
The oral clearance is 600mL/min, with about 7% by renal clearance.

Fig. 2.13 Absorption, distribution, metabolism, and excretion of escitalopram

2.2.5 What Is the Mechanism of Actions of Escitalopram?

The antidepressant mechanism of action of the S-enantiomer of citalopram, escitalopram, is considered to be associated with the serotonergic activity potentiation in the central nervous system (CNS) due to inhibition of CNS neuronal reuptake of serotonin (5-HT) (Fig. 2.14) [5].

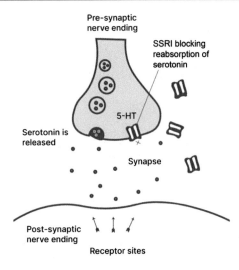

Fig. 2.14 Mechanism of actions of escitalopram

2.2.6 What Happens if Escitalopram Is Discontinued?

Abrupt discontinuation is not recommended with escitalopram, as abrupt cessation of these drugs is associated with a discontinuation syndrome. Therefore, the discontinuation of these drugs should be accomplished with gradual dose tapering [5].

2.2.7 What Are the Contraindications of Escitalopram?

Contraindications of Escitalopram (Fig. 2.15) [5].
What Are the Most Common or Most Worrisome Adverse Reactions Associated with Escitalopram (Fig. 2.16)?

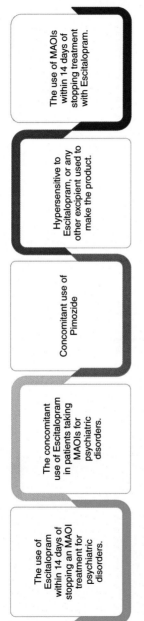

Fig. 2.15 Contraindications of escitalopram. MAOI: Monoamine oxidase inhibitor

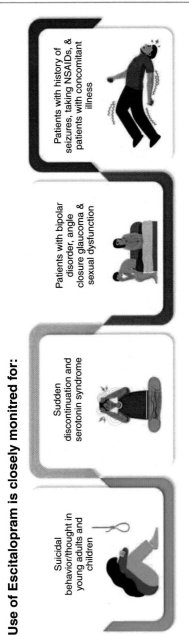

Fig. 2.16 Warning and precautions while using escitalopram

2.2.8 What Are the Most Common or Most Worrisome Adverse Reactions Associated with Escitalopram?

The most commonly noted adverse reactions of escitalopram include nausea, increased sweating, fatigue, insomnia, ejaculation disorder (primarily ejaculatory delay), drowsiness, anorgasmia, and decreased libido [5].

2.2.9 What Are the Clinically Important Drug Interactions Associated with Escitalopram?

Concomitant use of escitalopram with SSRIs, serotonin, norepinephrine reuptake inhibitors, or tryptophan is not recommended. It should be used with caution when concomitantly used with drugs affecting hemostasis [5].

Drugs that Interact with Escitalopram when Co-administered (Fig. 2.17) [5].

2.2.10 Use in Special Population (Fig. 2.18)?

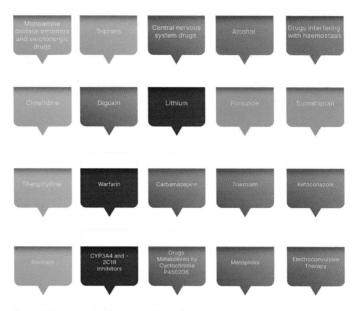

Fig. 2.17 Drugs that Interact with escitalopram when co-administered

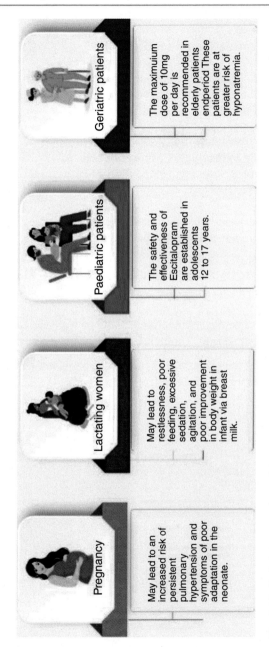

Fig. 2.18 Escitalopram use in special population

2.3   Fluoxetine

2.3.1   Introduction and Indications

Fluoxetine is a selective serotonin reuptake inhibitor (SSRI) approved by the United States Food and Drug Administration (USFDA) in 1987 [7].

Structure of fluoxetine (Fig. 2.19) [8].
What Are the Indications of Fluoxetine (Fig. 2.20)?
  In the United States, fluoxetine is an SSRI indicated for the treatment of [7, 8]:

- Acute and maintenance treatment of major depressive disorder (MDD) in adult and pediatric patients aged 8–18 years.
- Acute and maintenance treatment of obsessive-compulsive disorder (OCD) in adult and pediatric patients aged 7–17 years.
- Acute and maintenance treatment of bulimia nervosa in adult patients.
- Acute treatment of panic disorder, with or without agoraphobia, in adult patients.

  Fluoxetine and olanzapine in combination are indicated in the United States for (Fig. 2.21) [9]:

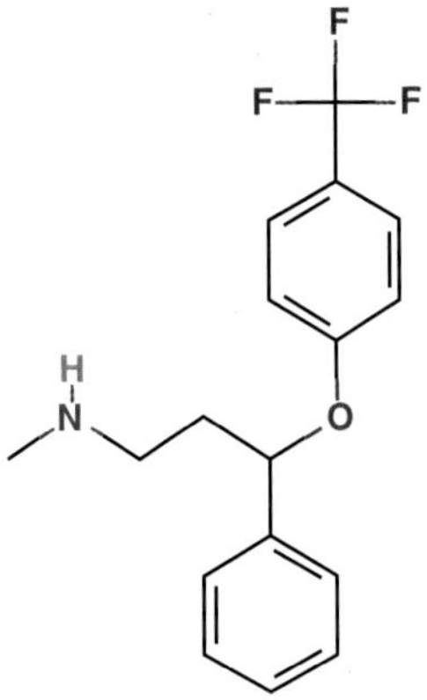

Fig. 2.19 Structure of
fluoxetine

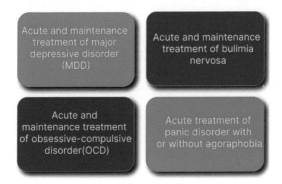

Fig. 2.20 Indications of fluoxetine

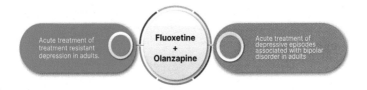

Fig. 2.21 Fluoxetine and olanzapine combination

- Acute treatment of depressive episodes associated with bipolar I disorder in adults.
- Acute treatment of treatment-resistant depression in adults (major depressive disorder in adult patients who do not respond to two separate trials of different antidepressants of adequate dose and duration in the current episode).

The indications of fluoxetine and the indications of its combination with olanzapine may be different in other countries.

2.3.2 What Are the Dosing Regimens for Fluoxetine?

Fluoxetine should be administered with or without food. The dosing regimen of fluoxetine varies based on the type of indication for which it is prescribed [7].

The Dosing Regimen for Fluoxetine: Based on the Indication (Fig. 2.22) [7].

The dose should be lowered, or the frequency of dosing should be reduced in patients with hepatic impairment, elderly patients, and patients with concurrent disease or on several concomitant medications [7].

When fluoxetine is used in combination with olanzapine [7]:

- Dose adjustments are required based on efficacy and tolerability.
- Monotherapy with Fluoxetine is not indicated to treat treatment-resistant depression or depressive episodes associated with bipolar I disorder.
- Safety in adults has not been evaluated for the concurrent use of doses above 18 mg olanzapine with 75 mg fluoxetine.
- Safety in children has not been evaluated for the concurrent use of doses above 12 mg olanzapine with 50 mg fluoxetine.

2.3.3   What Are the Pharmacokinetic Profiles of Fluoxetine?

Absorption, Distribution, Metabolism, and Excretion of Fluoxetine (Fig. 2.23) [7].

2.3.4   What Are the Pharmacodynamic Profiles of Fluoxetine?

Clinically relevant doses of fluoxetine block the serotonin uptake into human platelets as per the studies in humans. Animal studies also suggest that fluoxetine is a potent serotonin uptake inhibitor compared to norepinephrine [7].

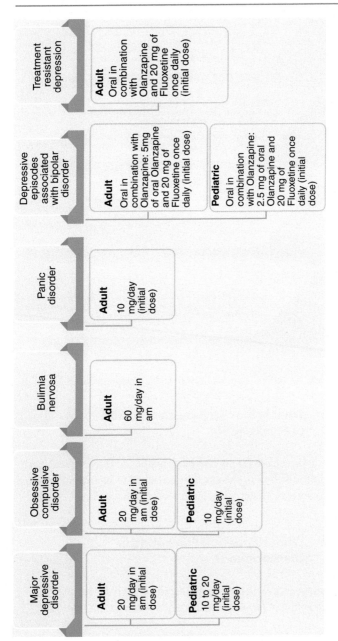

Fig. 2.22 The dosing regimen for fluoxetine

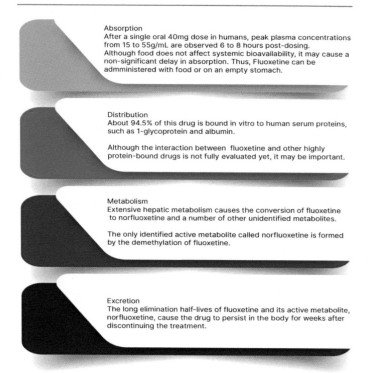

Absorption
After a single oral 40mg dose in humans, peak plasma concentrations from 15 to 55g/mL are observed 6 to 8 hours post-dosing. Although food does not affect systemic bioavailability, it may cause a non-significant delay in absorption. Thus, Fluoxetine can be admministered with food or on an empty stomach.

Distribution
About 94.5% of this drug is bound in vitro to human serum proteins, such as 1-glycoprotein and albumin.

Although the interaction between fluoxetine and other highly protein-bound drugs is not fully evaluated yet, it may be important.

Metabolism
Extensive hepatic metabolism causes the conversion of fluoxetine to norfluoxetine and a number of other unidentified metabolites.

The only identified active metabolite called norfluoxetine is formed by the demethylation of fluoxetine.

Excretion
The long elimination half-lives of fluoxetine and its active metabolite, norfluoxetine, cause the drug to persist in the body for weeks after discontinuing the treatment.

Fig. 2.23 Absorption, distribution, metabolism, and excretion of fluoxetine

2.3.5 What Is the Mechanism of Action of Fluoxetine?

The exact mechanism of fluoxetine is unknown. However, the mechanism of this drug is presumed to be linked to its inhibition of the central nervous system neuronal serotonin uptake (Fig. 2.24) [7].

2.3.6 What Happens if Fluoxetine Is Discontinued?

Adverse reactions upon discontinuation have been reported during the marketing of fluoxetine, particularly when abrupt (Fig. 2.25) [7].

Fig. 2.24 Mechanism of action of fluoxetine

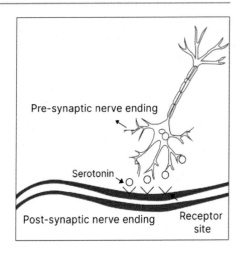

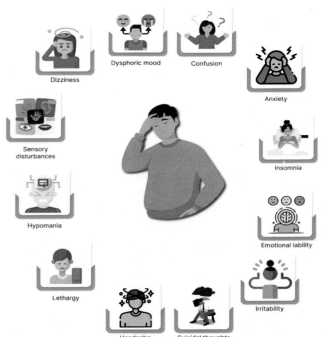

Fig. 2.25 Adverse reactions upon discontinuation of fluoxetine

Although these reactions are usually self-limiting, serious dis-continuation symptoms have also been reported. Thus, patients should be carefully monitored when discontinuing treatment [7].

A gradual reduction of dose is recommended whenever pos-sible.

Resuming the previously taken dose may be considered if intolerable symptoms occur after a dose reduction or upon treatment discontinuation.

Subsequently, a more gradual dose reduction should be considered [7].

2.3.7 What Are the Contraindications of Fluoxetine?

Contraindications of Fluoxetine (Fig. 2.26) [7].

2.3.8 What Are the Warnings and Precautions of Fluoxetine (Fig. 2.27)?

2.3.9 What Are the Most Common or Most Worrisome Adverse Reactions Associated with Fluoxetine (Fig. 2.28)?

Adverse reactions associated with fluoxetine [7, 9].

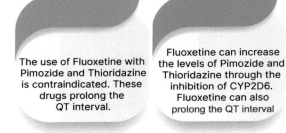

The use of Fluoxetine with Pimozide and Thioridazine is contraindicated. These drugs prolong the QT interval.

Fluoxetine can increase the levels of Pimozide and Thioridazine through the inhibition of CYP2D6. Fluoxetine can also prolong the QT interval

Fig. 2.26 Contraindications of fluoxetine

2.3.10 What Are the Clinically Important Drug Interactions Associated with Fluoxetine?

Drug interactions associated with fluoxetine (Table 2.3).

2.3.11 Use in Special Populations?

Fluoxetine in Pregnancy, Pediatric Population, and Hepatic Impairment (Fig. 2.29).

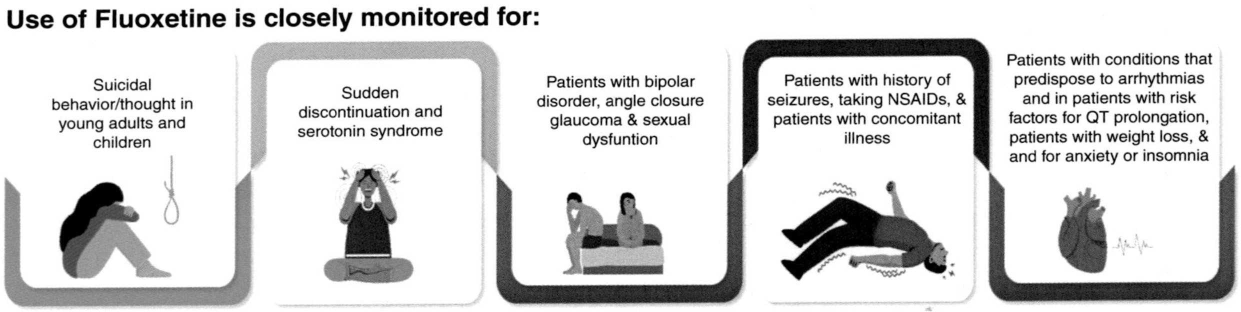

Use of Fluoxetine is closely monitored for:

Suicidal behavior/thought in young adults and children

Sudden discontinuation and serotonin syndrome

Patients with bipolar disorder, angle closure glaucoma & sexual dysfuntion

Patients with history of seizures, taking NSAIDs, & patients with concomitant illness

Patients with conditions that predispose to arrhythmias and in patients with risk factors for QT prolongation, patients with weight loss, & and for anxiety or insomnia

Fig. 2.27 Warnings and precautions of fluoxetine

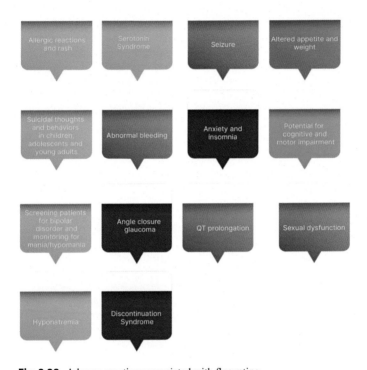

Fig. 2.28 Adverse reactions associated with fluoxetine

Table 2.3 Drug interactions associated with fluoxetine

Monoamine oxidase inhibitors (MAOIs):	It is contraindicated to use MAOIs for psychiatric disorders with fluoxetine or within 5 weeks of discontinuing fluoxetine due to the increased risk of serotonin syndrome
	It is contraindicated to use fluoxetine within 14 days of discontinuing MAOI used for psychiatric disorders
	Initiating fluoxetine in those treated with MAOIs, such as intravenous methylene blue or linezolid, is also contraindicated due to the increased risk of serotonin syndrome

(continued)

Table 2.3 (continued)

Serotonergic drugs:	Serotonin syndrome has been reported with SSRIs, including fluoxetine. It can occur when fluoxetine is taken alone but mainly when it is co-administered with other serotonergic agents, e.g., tryptophan, tricyclic antidepressants, fentanyl, triptans, and lithium. The treatment with fluoxetine should be discontinued if symptoms of serotonin syndrome are observed in patients. If concomitant use of fluoxetine with other serotonergic drugs is a clinical requirement, patients should be informed about the increased risk for serotonin syndrome, especially during treatment initiation and dose increases
Drugs metabolized by enzyme CYP2D6	Fluoxetine can potentially elevate the levels of haloperidol and clozapine
	Drugs that interfere with hemostasis (e.g., aspirin, warfarin, and NSAIDs) may potentiate bleeding risk
Tricyclic antidepressants (TCAs):	TCA levels should be monitored if co-administered with fluoxetine or when fluoxetine has been discontinued recently
	Drugs acting on the central nervous system: Exercise caution when fluoxetine is taken in combination with other centrally acting drugs
Antipsychotics	Fluoxetine can potentially elevate the levels of haloperidol and clozapine
Benzodiazepines	Diazepam increased 1%, alprazolam further psychomotor performance decrement due to increased levels
Anticonvulsants	Fluoxetine may lead to elevated levels of phenytoin and carbamazepine and clinical anticonvulsant toxicity
	Drugs tightly bound to plasma proteins: These drugs may cause a shift in plasma concentrations

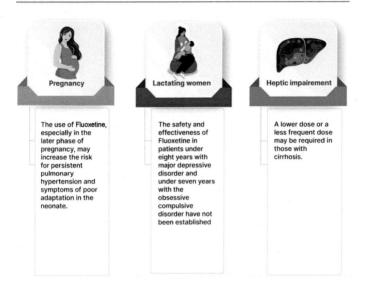

Fig. 2.29   Fluoxetine in pregnancy, pediatric population, and hepatic impairment

2.4   Fluvoxamine

2.4.1   Introduction and Indications

Fluvoxamine is classified as a selective serotonin reuptake inhibitor (SSRI). Fluvoxamine was first approved for marketing in Switzerland in 1983 after clinical trials for depression began in the 1970s. However, the United States approved fluvoxamine for treating obsessive-compulsive disorder (OCD) in the late 1980s [10].

Structure of Fluvoxamine (Fig. 2.30) [10].

Fluvoxamine is indicated in treating obsessive-compulsive disorder (OCD) in adults and children in the United States. In other countries, fluvoxamine is also indicated in treating depression (major depressive disorder) in adults [11].

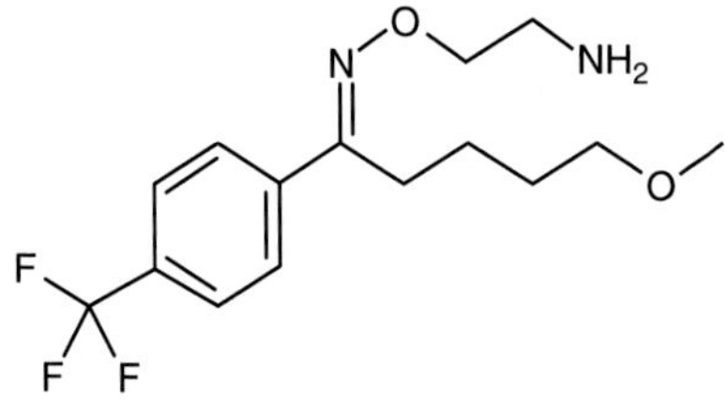

Fig. 2.30 Structure of
fluvoxamine

2.4.2 What Are the Dosing Regimens for Fluvoxamine? (Table 2.4) [11, 12]

Patients with renal or hepatic impairment and elderly patients should begin on low doses of fluvoxamine under close monitoring.

2.4.3 What Is the Pharmacokinetic Profile of Fluvoxamine?

Absorption, Distribution, Metabolism, and Excretion of Fluvoxamine (Fig. 2.31) [13].
Pharmacokinetics of Fluvoxamine in Patients with Hepatic and Renal Impairment (Fig. 2.32) [13].

2.4.4 What Is the Pharmacodynamic Profile of Fluvoxamine?

Fluvoxamine showed no significant affinity for dopaminergic, muscarinic, alpha beta-adrenergic, or histaminergic receptors in in vitro studies. It is suggested that the extrapyramidal, sedative, cardiovascular, and anticholinergic effects of certain psychiatric medications are related to antagonistic interactions with some of these receptors [12].

Table 2.4 Dosing regimens of fluvoxamine

Obsessive-compulsive disorder (OCD)	Depression (major depressive disorder)

• Adults:
  Recommended dose: ⊗ 100–300 mg daily.
  Initial dose: ⊗ 50 mg daily (with increases of 50 mg every 4–7 days as tolerated to maximum effect till the therapeutic response is achieved).
  Maximum dose: ⊗ should not exceed 300 mg in a day. Daily doses over 100 mg should be divided into two or three doses.
• Children (aged 8 years and above)
  Recommended dose: ⊗ 100 mg two times daily for 10 weeks.
  Initial dose: ⊗ 25 mg daily (with increases of 25 mg every 4–7 days as tolerated to maximum effect).
  Maximum dose: ⊗ should not exceed 200 mg/day (8–11 years) or 300 mg/day (12–17 years). Daily doses over 50 mg should be divided.
	• Adults:
	  Recommended dose: ⊗ 100 mg daily.
	  Initial dose: ⊗ 50 mg or 100 mg single dose daily at bed time (gradually can be increased till the therapeutic response is achieved).
	  Maximum dose: ⊗ should not exceed 300 mg in a day. A single dose up to 150 mg can be given in the evening time. Doses more than 150 mg should be divided in two or more doses.
	• Children (aged 8 years and above)
	  Fluvoxamine is not recommended to treat depression in children due to a lack of available data on its efficacy and safety.

2.4.5 What Is the Mechanism of Action of Fluvoxamine?

Fluvoxamine is thought to work by specifically inhibiting serotonin reuptake in brain neurons, in OCD. Fluvoxamine appears to be a more potent inhibitor of serotonin reuptake in vitro than fluoxetine, but not as potent as other SSRIs like paroxetine, sertraline, and citalopram, despite variations in published data [10].

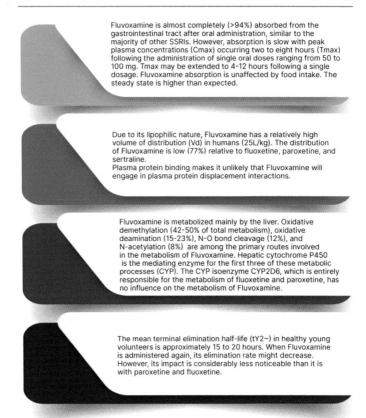

Fig. 2.31 Absorption, distribution, metabolism, and excretion of fluvoxamine

Fluvoxamine enhances the effects of serotonin on 5HT1A autoreceptors by blocking serotonin absorption at the sodium-dependent serotonin transporter (SERT) of the neuronal membrane. Fluvoxamine exhibits very little affinity for muscarinic, histamine H1, GABA-benzodiazepine, α1-, α2-, β-adrenergic, dopamine D2, opiate, 5-HT1, or 5-HT2 receptors [14].

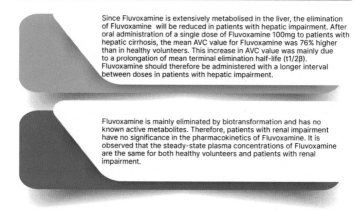

Since Fluvoxamine is extensively metabolised in the liver, the elimination of Fluvoxamine will be reduced in patients with hepatic impairment. After oral administration of a single dose of Fluvoxamine 100mg to patients with hepatic cirrhosis, the mean AVC value for Fluvoxamine was 76% higher than in healthy volunteers. This increase in AVC value was mainly due to a prolongation of mean terminal elimination half-life (t1/2β). Fluvoxamine should therefore be administered with a longer interval between doses in patients with hepatic impairment.

Fluvoxamine is mainly eliminated by biotransformation and has no known active metabolites. Therefore, patients with renal impairment have no significance in the pharmacokinetics of Fluvoxamine. It is observed that the steady-state plasma concentrations of Fluvoxamine are the same for both healthy volunteers and patients with renal impairment.

Fig. 2.32 Pharmacokinetic profile of fluvoxamine in patients with hepatic and renal impairment

2.4.6 What Happens if Fluvoxamine Is Discontinued [12] (Fig. 2.33)?

The following side effects, which have been routinely reported with fluvoxamine and other SSRIs and SNRIs (serotonin and norepinephrine reuptake inhibitors), occurred when these medications are stopped abruptly:

When discontinuing fluvoxamine, patients should be monitored for these symptoms. Whenever possible, it is advised to gradually lower the dosage instead of stopping suddenly. Resuming the previously prescribed dose may be considered if intolerable symptoms arise after a decrease in the dose or upon stopping the medication. The doctor may then decide to gradually reduce the dosage as needed.

2.4.7 What Are the Contraindications of Fluvoxamine?

Contraindications of Fluvoxamine (Fig. 2.34) [11, 12].

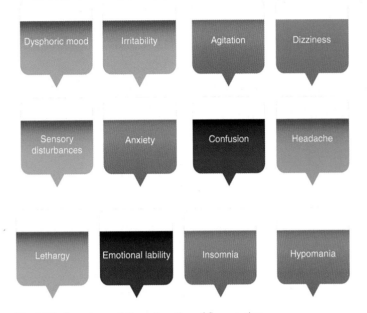

Fig. 2.33 Symptoms of discontinuation of fluvoxamine

2.4.8   What Are the Warnings and Precautions of Fluvoxamine [12] (Fig. 2.35)?

2.4.9   What Are the Most Common or Most Worrisome Adverse Reactions Associated with Fluvoxamine?

During various trials, fluvoxamine is well tolerated by patients. The safety and tolerability of fluvoxamine are the same as other SSRIs (citalopram and paroxetine) and have better antiobsessional properties than clomipramine. The adverse reactions associated with fluvoxamine are the same in both patients with depression and OCD (Fig. 2.36) [10, 12].

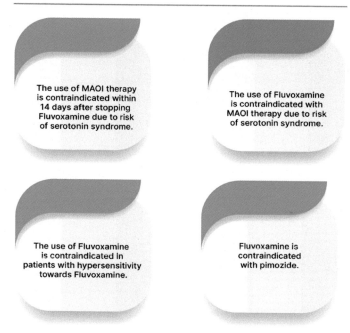

The use of MAOI therapy is contraindicated within 14 days after stopping Fluvoxamine due to risk of serotonin syndrome.

The use of Fluvoxamine is contraindicated with MAOI therapy due to risk of serotonin syndrome.

The use of Fluvoxamine is contraindicated in patients with hypersensitivity towards Fluvoxamine.

Fluvoxamine is contraindicated with pimozide.

Fig. 2.34 Contraindications of fluvoxamine. MAOI: Monoamine oxidase inhibitor

In children with OCD, the following adverse reactions are observed (Fig. 2.37) [12].

2.4.10 What Are the Clinically Important Drug Interactions Associated with Fluovoxamine [12] (Table 2.5)?

Overdose of Fluvoxamine (Fig. 2.38).

2.4.11 Use in Special Populations (Fig. 2.39) [12]?

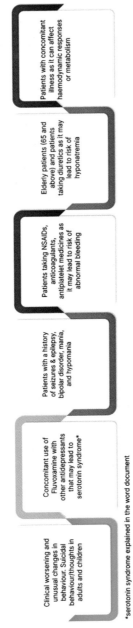

Clinical worsening and unusual changes in behaviour. Suicidal behaviour/thoughts in adults and children

Concomitant use of Fluvoxamine with other antidepressants that may lead to serotonin syndrome*

Patients with a history of seizures & epilepsy, bipolar disorder, mania, and hypomania

Patients taking NSAIDs, anticoagulants, antiplatelet medicines as it may lead to risk of abnormal bleeding

Elderly patients (65 and above) and patients taking diuretics as it may lead to risk of hyponatremia

Patients with concomitant illness as it can affect haemodynamic responses or metabolism

*serotonin syndrome explained in the word document

Fig. 2.35 Warning and precautions of fluvoxamine

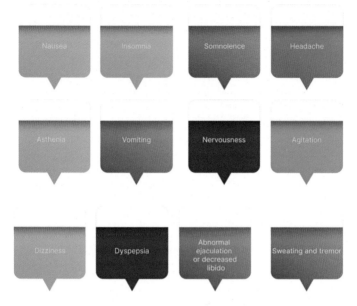

Fig. 2.36 Adverse reactions of fluvoxamine in adults

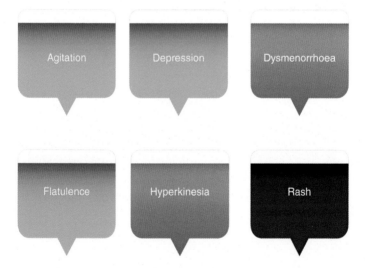

Fig. 2.37 Adverse reactions of fluvoxamine in children with OCD

Table 2.5 Drug interactions associated with fluvoxamine

Drugs that interact with cytochrome P450 isoenzymes	Fluvoxamine inhibits several types of cytochrome P450 isoenzymes, which are responsible for the metabolism of certain medicines including CYP1A2 (e.g., warfarin, theophylline, propranolol, tizanidine), CYP2C9 (e.g., warfarin), CYP3A4 (e.g., alprazolam), and CYP2C19 (e.g., omeprazole)
CNS active drugs	Significant declines in cognitive performance were seen with both lorazepam alone and lorazepam with fluvoxamine; however, the combined use of the two drugs did not result in greater mean decline than with lorazepam alone It is not recommended to take fluvoxamine with diazepam as fluvoxamine decreases the clearance of diazepam and N-desmethyldiazepam, its active metabolite fluvoxamine may decrease the clearance of benzodiazepines metabolized by hepatic oxidation, such as alprazolam, midazolam, triazolam, and so on. Therefore, these medications should be used cautiously Fluvoxamine with alprazolam tends to double the plasma concentration of alprazolam leading to decreased psychomotor performance and memory. Therefore, dose adjustment of alprazolam should be considered when administered along with fluvoxamine
Drugs that interfere with hemostasis (NSAIDs, antiplatelet, and anticoagulants)	Concomitant use of fluvoxamine with drugs, including NSAIDs, warfarin, aspirin, etc., should be monitored as psychotropic drugs interfere with serotonin uptake causing upper gastrointestinal bleeding
Theophylline and ramelteon	Fluvoxamine interferes with the clearance of theophylline. Therefore, theophylline dose should be reduced to one-third when co-administered with fluvoxamine. No need to change the dose of fluvoxamine. Fluvoxamine when administered with ramelteon results in increased plasma concentration of ramelteon; hence, it should not be given as a combination

(continued)

Table 2.5 (continued)

Other serotonergic agents (TCAs, triptans, etc.)	Fluvoxamine tends to increase the plasma concentration of TCAS and might have risk of serotonin syndrome when used with triptans. Therefore, the combination of fluvoxamine with TCAs and triptans should be carefully monitored
Thioridazine and pimozide	Administration of fluvoxamine and thioridazine combination causes prolongation of QTc prolongation which is dose-related. It is further linked to significant ventricular arrhythmias, including torsades de pointes-type arrhythmias as well as sudden death. The cytochrome P4503A4 isoenzyme is responsible for the metabolism of pimozide. Research has shown that ketoconazole, a strong inhibitor of CYP3A4, prevents this drug's metabolism, leading to elevated levels of the parent drug in the plasma. Increased pimozide plasma concentrations have been linked to torsades de pointes-type ventricular tachycardia that might be fatal as well as QT prolongation. Hence fluvoxamine and pimozide combination is not recommended

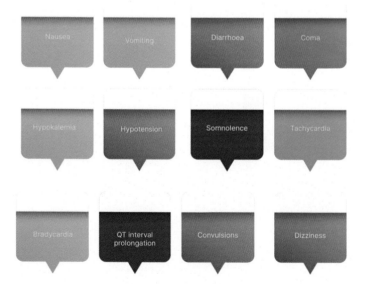

Fig. 2.38 Symptoms of fluvoxamine overdose

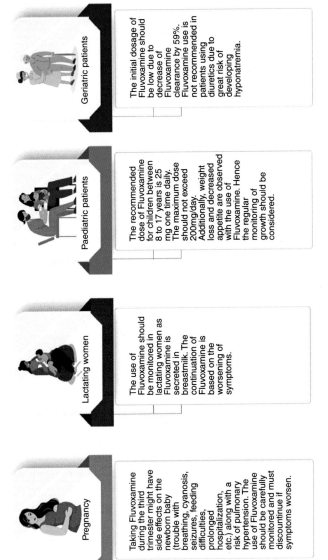

Fig. 2.39 Fluvoxamine in special populations

Geriatric patients

The initial dosage of Fluvoxamine should be low due to decrease of Fluvoxamine clearance by 59%. Fluvoxamine use is not recommended in patients using diuretics due to great risk of developing hyponatremia.

Paediatric patients

The recommended dose of Fluvoxamine for children between 8 to 17 years is 25 mg one time daily. The maximum dose should not exceed 200mg/day. Additionally, weight loss and decreased appetite are observed with the use of Fluvoxamine. Hence the regular monitoring of growth should be considered.

Lactating women

The use of Fluvoxamine should be monitored in lactating women as Fluvoxamine is secreted in breastmilk. The continuation of Fluvoxamine is based on the worsening of symptoms.

Pregnancy

Taking Fluvoxamine during the third trimester might have side effects on the newborn baby (trouble with breathing, cyanosis, seizures, feeding difficulties, prolonged hospitalization, etc.) along with a risk of pulmonary hypertension. The use of Fluvoxamine should be carefully monitored and must discountinue if symptoms worsen.

2.5   Paroxetine

2.5.1   Introduction and Indications

Paroxetine is a selective serotonin reuptake inhibitor (SSRI), which was initially approved by the United States Food and Drug Administration in 1992.

Structure of Paroxetine (Fig. 2.40).
What Are the Indications of Paroxetine (Fig. 2.41)?

In the United States, paroxetine is indicated for the treatment of the following conditions [15, 16, 2].

The indications may be different in other countries.

2.5.2   What Are the Dosing Regimens for Paroxetine?

Paroxetine should be administered once daily in the morning, with or without food. The dose of paroxetine should be reduced gradually while discontinuing the treatment [15].

The Dosing Regimen for Paroxetine: Based on Indication (Fig. 2.42 and Table 2.6) [15].

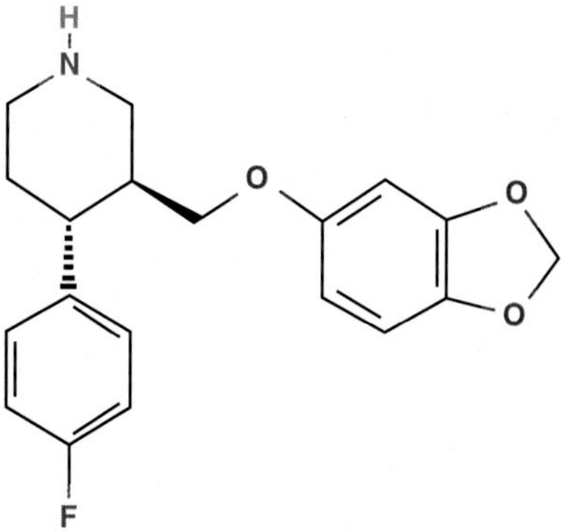

Fig. 2.40 Structure of paroxetine

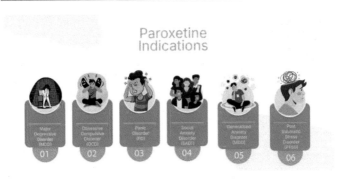

Fig. 2.41 Paroxetine indications

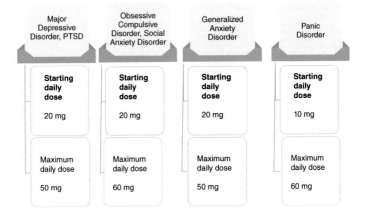

Fig. 2.42 The dosing regimen for paroxetine

Table 2.6 The dosing regimen for paroxetine

Indication	Starting daily dose	Maximum daily dose
MDD	20 mg	50 mg
OCD	20 mg	60 mg
PD	10 mg	60 mg
PTSD	20 mg	50 mg

In elderly patients and patients with severe renal or hepatic impairment, the starting dose is 10 mg/day, and the maximum dose is 40 mg/day [15].

2.5.3 What Are the Pharmacokinetic Profiles of Paroxetine?

Absorption, Distribution, Metabolism, and Excretion of Paroxetine (Fig. 2.43) [15].

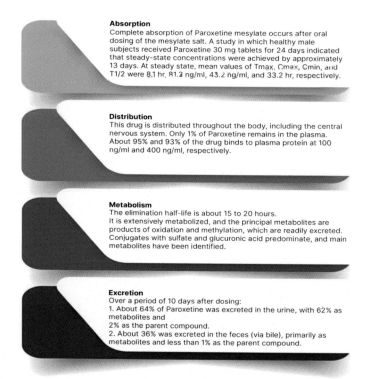

Absorption
Complete absorption of Paroxetine mesylate occurs after oral dosing of the mesylate salt. A study in which healthy male subjects received Paroxetine 30 mg tablets for 24 days indicated that steady-state concentrations were achieved by approximately 13 days. At steady state, mean values of Tmax, Cmax, Cmin, and T1/2 were 8.1 hr, 81.3 ng/ml, 43.2 ng/ml, and 33.2 hr, respectively.

Distribution
This drug is distributed throughout the body, including the central nervous system. Only 1% of Paroxetine remains in the plasma. About 95% and 93% of the drug binds to plasma protein at 100 ng/ml and 400 ng/ml, respectively.

Metabolism
The elimination half-life is about 15 to 20 hours.
It is extensively metabolized, and the principal metabolites are products of oxidation and methylation, which are readily excreted. Conjugates with sulfate and glucuronic acid predominate, and main metabolites have been identified.

Excretion
Over a period of 10 days after dosing:
1. About 64% of Paroxetine was excreted in the urine, with 62% as metabolites and
2% as the parent compound.
2. About 36% was excreted in the feces (via bile), primarily as metabolites and less than 1% as the parent compound.

Fig. 2.43 Absorption, distribution, metabolism, and excretion of paroxetine. C_{max}: Peak plasma concentration; T_{max}: Time to reach C_{max}

2.5.4   What Are the Pharmacodynamic Profiles of Paroxetine?

As per the studies performed with clinically relevant doses of paroxetine in humans, paroxetine blocks serotonin uptake into human platelets. In vitro animal studies suggest that this drug is a potent and highly selective neuronal serotonin reuptake inhibitor with only feeble effects on neuronal norepinephrine and dopamine reuptake [15].

2.5.5   What Is the Mechanism of Actions of Paroxetine (Fig. 2.44)?

Although the mechanism of action of paroxetine in treating MDD, OCD, PD, and GAD is not known, it is presumed to be associated with potentiating serotonergic activity in the central nervous system due to the inhibition of neuronal reuptake of serotonin [15].

2.5.6   What Happens if Paroxetine Is Discontinued (Fig. 2.45)?

Discontinuing paroxetine, especially abruptly discontinuing paroxetine, leads to adverse reactions, such as sweating, nausea, dys-

Fig. 2.44 Mechanism of actions of paroxetine

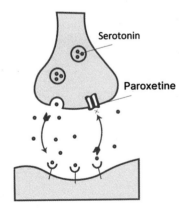

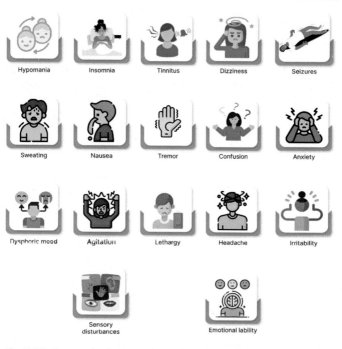

Fig. 2.45 Symptoms of paroxetine discontinuation syndrome

phoric mood, agitation, anxiety, confusion, irritability, dizziness, tremor, sensory disturbances, headache, insomnia, hypomania, lethargy, emotional lability, seizures, and tinnitus. Therefore, a gradual dose reduction is recommended whenever possible [15].

Adverse reactions related to the discontinuation of paroxetine have also been reported in pediatric patients. The safety and effectiveness of paroxetine in children are not established [15].

2.5.7 What Are the Contraindications of Paroxetine?

Due to the risk of serotonin syndrome, all serotonergic medications are contraindicated with MAOIs [15].

Contraindications of Paroxetine (Fig. 2.46) [15].

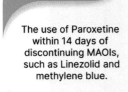

The use of Paroxetine within 14 days of discontinuing MAOIs, such as Linezolid and methylene blue.

Known hypersensitivity, such as anaphylaxis, angioedema, or Stevens-Johnson syndrome, to Paroxetine or to any of the inactive ingredients in the product

Fig. 2.46 Contraindications of paroxetine. MAOI: Monoamine oxidase inhibitor

2.5.8 What Are the Warnings and Precautions of Paroxetine?

The warnings and precautions for patients using paroxetine include the following (Fig. 2.47) [15]:

- **Serotonin syndrome:** Patients are at increased risk of serotonin syndrome when paroxetine is co-administered with other serotonergic agents and when taken alone. If it occurs, paroxetine should be discontinued, and supportive measures should be initiated.
- **Embryofetal and neonatal toxicity:** Paroxetine can harm the fetus and neonates. If the mother is exposed to paroxetine during the first trimester, there is an increased risk of cardiovascular malformations. However, exposure in late pregnancy increases the risk for persistent pulmonary hypertension in newborns.
- **Increased risk of bleeding:** The risk of bleeding increases due to the concurrent use of certain drugs with paroxetine. These drugs include nonsteroidal anti-inflammatory, antiplatelet, and anticoagulant drugs.

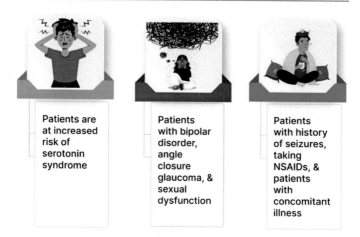

| Patients are at increased risk of serotonin syndrome | Patients with bipolar disorder, angle closure glaucoma, & sexual dysfunction | Patients with history of seizures, taking NSAIDs, & patients with concomitant illness |

Fig. 2.47 Warnings and precautions of paroxetine

- **Activation of mania/hypomania:** Patients should be evaluated to check if they have bipolar disorder.
- **Seizures:** Paroxetine should be used with caution in patients with seizure disorders.
- **Angle-closure glaucoma:** Patients with untreated anatomically narrow angles are at risk of developing angle-closure glaucoma when treated with antidepressants.
- **Sexual dysfunction:** Paroxetine may lead to sexual dysfunction symptoms.

2.5.9 What Are the Most Common or Most Worrisome Adverse Reactions Associated with Paroxetine?

The most common adverse reactions ($\geq 5\%$ and at least twice placebo) of paroxetine include sweating, constipation, drowsiness, dizziness, insomnia, nausea, asthenia, decreased appetite, dry mouth, tremor, nervousness, libido decreased, ejaculatory

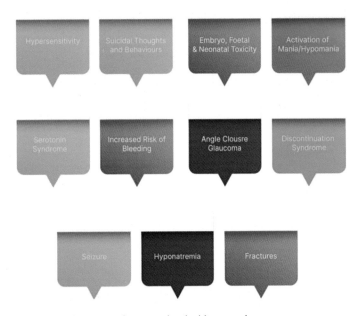

Fig. 2.48 Adverse reactions associated with paroxetine

disturbance, female genital disorders, impotence, other male genital disorders, infection, and orgasmic disturbance [15, 17].

Paroxetine is linked with a higher incidence of sexual dysfunction and more weight gain than other SSRIs [17, 18].

Adverse reactions associated with paroxetine (Fig. 2.48) [15].

2.5.10 What Are the Clinically Important Drug Interactions Associated with Paroxetine? (Table 2.7) [15, 16]

2.5.11 Use in Special Populations (Fig. 2.49)?

Table 2.7 Clinically important drug interactions associated with paroxetine

Monoamine oxidase inhibitors (MAOI)	The concomitant use of paroxetine with MAOIs increases the risk of serotonin syndrome. Concomitant use of paroxetine is contraindicated with an MAOI, such as intravenous methylene blue or linezolid, intended to treat psychiatric disorders. Examples of MAOIs: are phenelzine, selegiline, isocarboxazid, tranylcypromine, linezolid, and methylene blue
Pimozide and thioridazine [15]	Concomitant use of paroxetine with pimozide or thioridazine increases the plasma concentrations of pimozide and thioridazine. It may increase the risk of QTc prolongation and ventricular arrhythmias. Paroxetine is contraindicated in those on pimozide or thioridazine therapy
Other serotonergic drugs [15]	The risk of serotonin syndrome increases with the use of other serotonergic drugs. Patients should be monitored during treatment initiations and while uptitrating the dose. Paroxetine should be discontinued in case of any symptoms of serotonin syndrome. Examples of other serotonergic drugs include other SSRIs, triptans, SNRIs, fentanyl, lithium, tricyclic antidepressants, tramadol, St. John's wort, tryptophan, and buspirone
Drugs interfering with hemostasis [15]	The concomitant use of anticoagulants and antiplatelets with paroxetine may lead to an increased risk of bleeding. Patients should be informed about this, and the international normalized ratio should be monitored in these patients. Examples of antiplatelets and anticoagulants include heparin, clopidogrel, warfarin, and aspirin

(continued)

Table 2.7 (continued)

Drugs are highly bound to plasma protein [15]	Paroxetine is highly bound to plasma proteins. The concomitant use of other medications highly bound to plasma proteins may increase the free concentration of paroxetine or other highly bound medicines in the plasma. Example: Warfarin
Benzodiazepines	Diazepam—Increased t%, alprazolam—Further psychomotor performance decrement due to increased levels
Fosamprenavir/ritonavir [15]	Plasma levels of paroxetine are reduced when co-administered with fosamprenavir/ritonavir. Thus, dose adjustment may be required
Tamoxifen [15, 18]	Paroxetine, when co-administered with tamoxifen, may reduce the efficacy of tamoxifen. Thus, other antidepressant drugs with little or no effects on CYP2D6 should be considered
Drugs metabolized by CYP2D6 [15, 17]	Paroxetine is an inhibitor of CYP2D6. It may lead to an increase in the exposure of the CYP2D6 substrate. It is recommended to reduce the dose of CYP2D6 substrate if required. Examples of CYP2D6 substrates are flecainide, atomoxetine, propafenone, perphenazine, tolterodine, desipramine, dextromethorphan, metoprolol, risperidone, nebivolol, venlafaxine

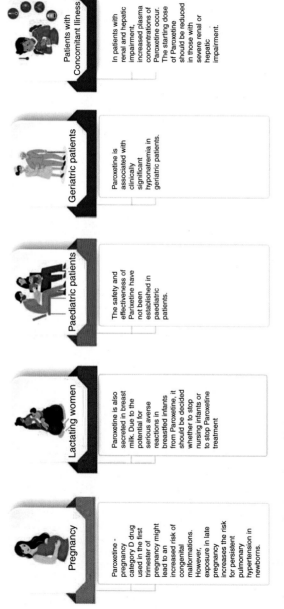

Fig. 2.49 Paroxetine in special populations

2.6   Sertraline

2.6.1   Introduction and Indications

Sertraline received its initial approval from the United States Food and Drug Administration in 1991 (Fig. 2.50) [18].

In the United States, Sertraline is indicated for the treatment of the following conditions (Fig. 2.51) [18]:

The indications may be different in other countries.

2.6.2   What Are the Dosing Regimens for Sertraline?

Sertraline can be administered with or without food. The dose of sertraline should be reduced gradually while discontinuing the treatment [18].

The Dosing Regimen in Patients with Hepatic Impairment (Fig. 2.52) [18].

The Dosing Regimen for Sertraline: Based on Indication (Fig. 2.53 **and** Table 2.8) [18].

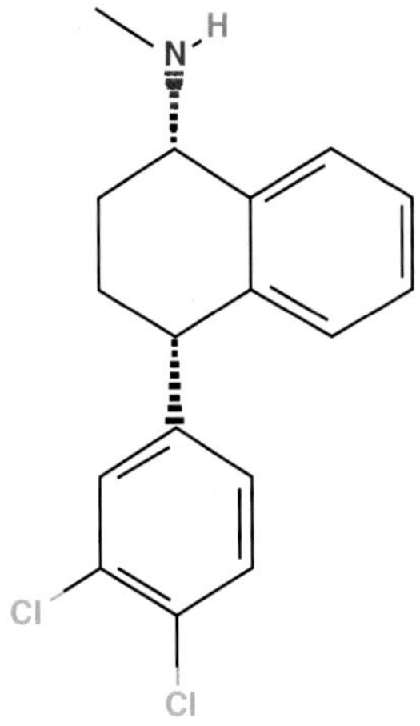

Fig. 2.50 Structure of sertraline

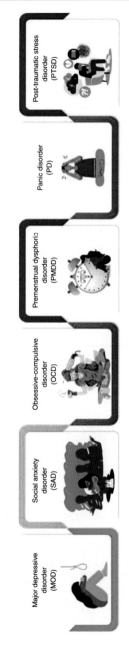

Fig. 2.51 Indications of sertraline

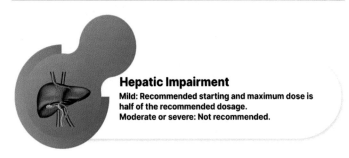

Hepatic Impairment
Mild: Recommended starting and maximum dose is half of the recommended dosage.
Moderate or severe: Not recommended.

Fig. 2.52 Dosing regimen in patients with hepatic impairment

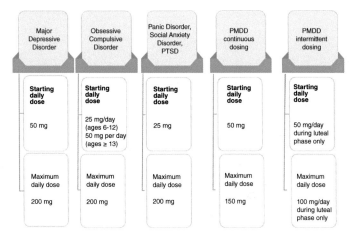

Major Depressive Disorder	Obsessive Compulsive Disorder	Panic Disorder, Social Anxiety Disorder, PTSD	PMDD continuous dosing	PMDD intermittent dosing
Starting daily dose	**Starting daily dose**	**Starting daily dose**	**Starting daily dose**	**Starting daily dose**
50 mg	25 mg/day (ages 6-12) 50 mg per day (ages ≥ 13)	25 mg	50 mg	50 mg/day during luteal phase only
Maximum daily dose	**Maximum daily dose**	**Maximum daily dose**	**Maximum daily dose**	**Maximum daily dose**
200 mg	200 mg	200 mg	150 mg	100 mg/day during luteal phase only

Fig. 2.53 The dosing regimen for sertraline. MDD: Major depressive disorder; OCD: Obsessive-compulsive disorder; PD: Panic disorder; PMDD: Premenstrual dysphoric disorder; PTSD: Post-traumatic stress disorder; SAD: Social anxiety disorder

In case of inadequate response to the starting dose of sertraline, titrate in 25–50 mg/day increments once weekly in MDD, PD, SAD, OCD, and PTSD.

The recommended starting dose of sertraline for treating PMDD in adult women is 50 mg/day. During a menstrual cycle, sertraline may be administered continuously, i.e., every day, or intermittently, i.e., only during the luteal phase [18].

Table 2.8 Indications and dosing regimen for sertraline

Indication	Starting dosage	Maximum dosage
Major depressive disorder (MDD).	50 mg per day	200 mg per day
Obsessive-compulsive disorder (OCD).	25 mg per day (ages 6–12), 50 mg per day (ages ≥13)	200 mg per day
Panic disorder (PD). Post-traumatic stress disorder (PTSD). Social anxiety disorder (SAD).	25 mg per day	200 mg per day
Premenstrual dysphoric disorder (PMDD) continuous dosing.	50 mg per day	150 mg per day
Premenstrual dysphoric disorder (PMDD) intermittent dosing.	50 mg per day during luteal phase only	100 mg per day during luteal phase only

- Women not responding to 50 mg/day of continuous dosing may benefit from increasing the dose at 50 mg increments during each menstrual cycle up to 150 mg/day.
- Women not responding to 50 mg/day of intermittent dosing may benefit from increasing the dose up to a maximum dose of 100 mg/day during the next menstrual cycle and all subsequent cycles as follows:
  - 50 mg/day during the first three dosing days, followed by 100 mg/day during the other days in the dosing cycle [18].

2.6.3   What Are the Pharmacokinetic Profiles of Sertraline?

Among the SSRIs, citalopram, escitalopram, and sertraline are the best tolerated and the ones with the least possibility of causing serious pharmacokinetic interactions [4].

Pharmacokinetic Profile of Sertraline (Fig. 2.54) [18]**.**

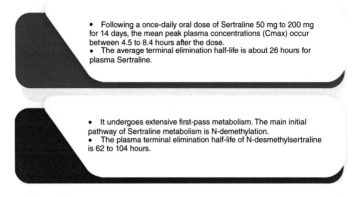

- Following a once-daily oral dose of Sertraline 50 mg to 200 mg for 14 days, the mean peak plasma concentrations (Cmax) occur between 4.5 to 8.4 hours after the dose.
- The average terminal elimination half-life is about 26 hours for plasma Sertraline.

- It undergoes extensive first-pass metabolism. The main initial pathway of Sertraline metabolism is N-demethylation.
- The plasma terminal elimination half-life of N-desmethylsertraline is 62 to 104 hours.

Fig. 2.54 Pharmacokinetic profile of sertraline

2.6.4   What Is the Mechanism of Actions of Sertraline?

Mechanism of Action of Sertraline (Fig. 2.55)**.**

Sertraline leads to potentiation of serotonergic activity in the central nervous system by inhibiting the neuronal reuptake of serotonin [18].

2.6.5   What Happens if Sertraline Is Discontinued?

Discontinuing sertraline can lead to adverse reactions. Thus, whenever possible, gradually reducing the dose of sertraline is recommended rather than abrupt discontinuation [18].

2.6.6   What Are the Contraindications of Sertraline?

Due to the risk of serotonin syndrome, all serotonergic medications are contraindicated with sertraline [18].

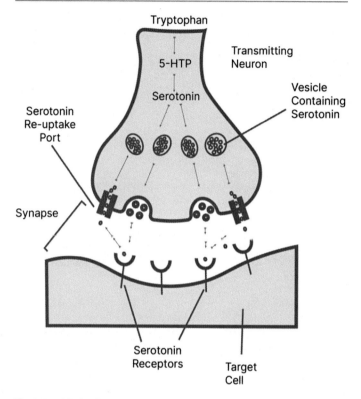

Fig. 2.55 Mechanism of action of sertraline

Contraindications of Sertraline (Fig. 2.56) [18].

2.6.7   What Are the Warnings and Precautions of Sertraline?

Warnings and Precautions for Patients Using Sertraline (Fig. 2.57) [18].

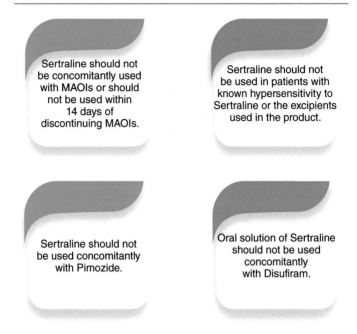

Fig. 2.56 Contraindications of sertraline. MAOI: Monoamine oxidase inhibitor

2.6.8 What Are the Most Common and Most Worrisome Adverse Reactions Associated with Sertraline?

Most common adverse reactions, i.e., >5% and twice placebo, of sertraline in pooled placebo-controlled MDD, OCD, PD, PTSD, SAD, and PMDD clinical trials included nausea, dyspepsia, diarrhea, tremor, ejaculation failure, decreased appetite, decreased libido, and hyperhidrosis [18].

Sertraline leads to a higher incidence of diarrhea as compared to other SSRIs [17].

Adverse reactions associated with sertraline (Fig. 2.58) [18].

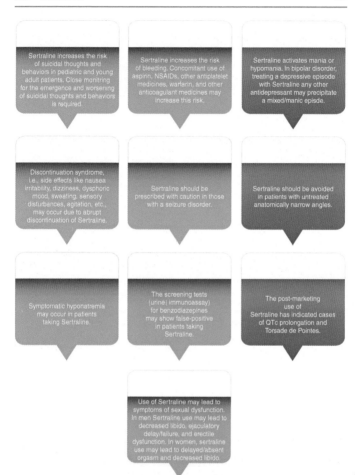

Fig. 2.57 Warnings and precautions for patients using sertraline. AIDS: Nonsteroidal anti-inflammatory drugs

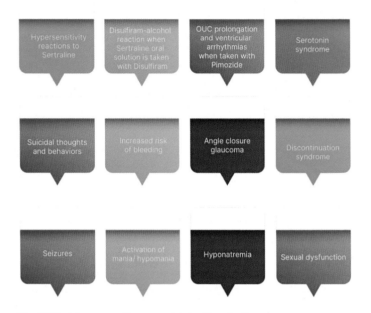

Fig. 2.58 Adverse reactions associated with sertraline

2.6.9 What Are the Clinically Important Drug Interactions Associated with Sertraline? (Table 2.9)

2.6.10 What Happens After Sertraline Overdose? How to Manage Sertraline Overdose?

Sertraline overdose (Fig. 2.59) [18].
Management of Sertraline Overdose [18].

Gastrointestinal decontamination using activated charcoal should be considered in those who present early after an overdose of sertraline.

Table 2.9 Clinically important drug interactions associated with sertraline

Monoamine oxidase inhibitors (MAOIs)	The concomitant use of sertraline with MAOIs increases the risk of serotonin syndrome. Concomitant use of sertraline is contraindicated in patients taking MAOIs, such as linezolid or intravenous methylene blue. Examples of MAOIs: tranylcypromine, selegiline, isocarboxazid, linezolid, and methylene blue
Other serotonergic drugs	Concomitant use of sertraline with other serotonergic drugs increases the risk of serotonin syndrome. Monitor for symptoms of serotonin syndrome, especially during initiation of treatment or dose titration. Discontinue the treatment if it occurs. Examples of other serotonergic drugs: Other SSRIs, SNRIs, triptans, tricyclic antidepressants, buspirone, lithium, tramadol, amphetamines, fentanyl, St. John's wort, and tryptophan
Drugs that interfere with hemostasis (antiplatelet agents and anticoagulants)	The concomitant use of sertraline with an antiplatelet agent may potentiate the bleeding risk. Patients at an increased risk of bleeding associated with the concomitant use of sertraline with antiplatelet agents and anticoagulants should be informed about it. For patients on warfarin therapy, the international normalized ratio should be carefully monitored. Examples of antiplatelets and anticoagulants: Clopidogrel, aspirin, heparin, and warfarin
Drugs highly bound to plasma protein	Sertraline is highly bound to plasma protein. The concurrent use of sertraline with other drugs highly bound to plasma protein may lead to increased free concentrations of sertraline or other tightly bound drugs in plasma. Monitor for side effects and reduce the dosage of sertraline or other protein-bound medications as warranted. Examples: Warfarin
Drugs metabolized by CYP2D6	Sertraline is an inhibitor of the enzyme CYP2D6. The concurrent use of sertraline with a CYP2D6 substrate may cause an increase in the exposure of the CYP2D6 substrate. It is recommended to reduce the dose of a CYP2D6 substrate if needed with concomitant sertraline use. On the contrary, an increase in the dose of a CYP2D6 substrate may be required if sertraline is discontinued. Examples of drugs metabolized by CYP2D6: Propafenone, atomoxetine, desipramine, metoprolol, flecainide, nebivolol, perphenazine, tolterodine, dextromethorphan, thioridazine, and venlafaxine

(continued)

Table 2.9 (continued)

Phenytoin	Phenytoin is a drug with a narrow therapeutic index. Sertraline may increase the concentration of phenytoin. It is recommended to monitor phenytoin levels when initiating or titrating sertraline. Phenytoin dose should be reduced if required. Examples: Fosphenytoin and phenytoin
Drugs that prolong the QTc interval	The risk of QTc prolongation and/or ventricular arrhythmias increases with concomitant use of other drugs which prolong the QTC interval. Examples of drugs that prolong QTc interval: Specific antibiotics (e.g., moxifloxacin, erythromycin, sparfloxacin, gatifloxacin); specific antipsychotics (e.g., ziprasidone, chlorpromazine, droperidol, iloperidone, mesoridazine); class 1A antiarrhythmic medications (e.g., quinidine, procainamide); class II antiarrhythmics (e.g., sotalol, amiodarone); and others (e.g., dolasetron mesylate, pentamidine, methadone, levomethadyl acetate, halofantrine, mefloquine, probucol, or tacrolimus)

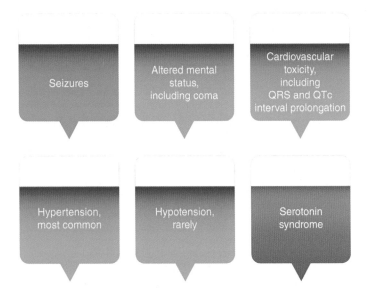

Fig. 2.59 Symptoms of sertraline overdose

2.6.11 Can Sertraline Be Prescribed to Special Populations? (Fig. 2.60)

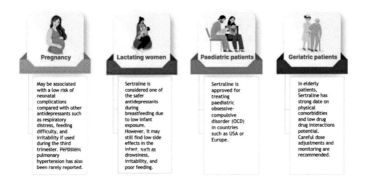

Pregnancy	Lactating women	Paediatric patients	Geriatric patients
May be associated with a low risk of neonatal complications compared with other antidepressants such as respiratory distress, feeding difficulty, and irritability if used during the third trimester. Persistent pulmonary hypertension has also been rarely reported.	Sertraline is considered one of the safer antidepressants during breastfeeding due to low infant exposure. However, it may still find low side effects in the infant, such as drowsiness, irritability, and poor feeding.	Sertraline is approved for treating paediatric obsessive-compulsive disorder (OCD) in countries such as USA or Europe.	In elderly patients, Sertraline has strong date on physical comorbidities and low drug drug interactions potential. Careful dose adjustments and monitoring are recommended.

Fig. 2.60 Sertraline in special populations

References

1. Sharbaf Shoar N, Fariba KA, Padhy RK. Citalopram. In: StatPearls [internet]. Treasure Island, FL: StatPearls Publishing; 2023 Nov 7. 2025 Jan–.
2. The United States Food and Drug Administration. Highlights of prescribing information. CELEXA (citalopram) tablets, for oral use. Updated 10/2023. Available from: https://www.accessdata.fda.gov/drugsatfda_docs/label/2024/020822s055lbl.pdf#page=22.
3. National Library of Medicine. Citalopram. Available from: https://pubchem.ncbi.nlm.nih.gov/compound/Citalopram#section=2D-Structure. Accessed on Feb 27, 2023.
4. McCarrell JL, Bailey TA, Duncan NA, Covington LP, Clifford KM, Hall RG, Blaszczyk AT. A review of citalopram dose restrictions in the treatment of neuropsychiatric disorders in older adults. Ment Health Clin. 2019;9(4):280–6. https://doi.org/10.9740/mhc.2019.07.280.
5. The United States Food and Drug Administration. Highlights of prescribing information. Lexapro® (Escitalopram) tablets and oral solution. Updated 04/2024. Available from: https://www.accessdata.fda.gov/drugsatfda_docs/label/2024/021323s058lbl.pdf.

6. National Library of Medicine. Escitalopram. Available from: https://pub-chem.ncbi.nlm.nih.gov/compound/Escitalopram. Accessed on Feb 28, 2023.

7. The United States Food and Drug Administration. Highlights of prescribing information. PROZAC (fluoxetine capsules) for oral use. Updated 08/2023. Available from: https://www.accessdata.fda.gov/drugsatfda_docs/label/2023/018936%20s112lbl.pdf.

8. National Library of Medicine. Fluoxetine. Available from: https://pub-chem.ncbi.nlm.nih.gov/compound/Fluoxetine. Accessed on Feb 09, 2023.

9. Fluoxetine and Olanzapine, prescribing information. Updated 08/2023. Available from: https://www.accessdata.fda.gov/drugsatfda_docs/label/2023/021520s055lbl.pdf.

10. Dell'Osso B, Allen A, Hollander E. Fluvoxamine: a selective serotonin re-uptake inhibitor for the treatment of obsessive-compulsive disorder. Expert Opin Pharmacother. 2005;6(15):2727–40. https://doi.org/10.1517/14656566.6.15.2727. PMID: 16316311. https://pubmed.ncbi.nlm.nih.gov/16316311/.

11. Fluvoxamine. [Internet]. [cited 2024 Mar 21]. Available from: https://www.medicines.org.uk/emc/product/1169/smpc#gref.

12. The United States Food and Drug Administration. Highlights of prescribing information. Luvox (Fluvoxamine) tablets, for oral use. Updated 08/2023. Available from: https://www.accessdata.fda.gov/drugsatfda_docs/label/2023/021519s026lbl.pdf.

13. van Harten J. Overview of the pharmacokinetics of fluvoxamine. Clin Pharmacokinet. 1995;29(Suppl 1):1–9. https://doi.org/10.2165/00003088-199500291-00003. PMID: 8846617. https://pubmed.ncbi.nlm.nih.gov/8846617/.

14. Sukhatme VP, Reiersen AM, Vayttaden SJ, Sukhatme VV. Fluvoxamine: a review of its mechanism of action and its role in COVID-19. Front Pharmacol. 2021;12:652688. https://www.frontiersin.org/journals/pharmacology/articles/10.3389/fphar.2021.652688/full.

15. The United States Food and Drug Administration. Highlights of prescribing information. Paxil tablets. Updated 02/2021. Available from: https://www.accessdata.fda.gov/drugsatfda_docs/label/2021/020031s077lbl.pdf.

16. The United States Food and Drug Administration. Highlights of prescribing information. BRISDELLE® (paroxetine) capsules. Updated 08/2023. Available from: https://www.accessdata.fda.gov/drugsatfda_docs/label/2023/020031s082lbl.pdf.

17. Liao Y, Sun Y, Guo J, Kang Z, Sun Y, Zhang Y, He J, Huang C, Sun X, Zhang J-M, Wang J, Wang H-N, Chen Z-Y, Wang K, Pan J, Ni A-H, Weng S, Wang A, Cao C, Sun L, Zhang Y, Kuang L, Zhang Y, Liu Z, Yue W,

Precision Medicine to Enhance Depression and Anxiety Outcome Consortium. Dose adjustment of paroxetine based on CYP2D6 activity score inferred metabolizer status in Chinese Han patients with depressive or anxiety disorders: a prospective study and cross-ethnic meta-analysis. EBioMedicine. 2024;104:105165. https://doi.org/10.1016/j.ebiom.2024.105165.

18. Edinoff AN, Akuly HA, Hanna TA, Ochoa CO, Patti SJ, Ghaffar YA, Kaye AD, Viswanath O, Urits I, Boyer AG, Cornett EM, Kaye AM. Selective serotonin reuptake inhibitors and adverse effects: a narrative review. Neurol Int. 2021, Aug 5;13(3):387–401. https://doi.org/10.3390/neurolint13030038. PMID: 34449705; PMCID: PMC8395812

SNRIs

3

3.1 Venlafaxine and Desvenlafaxine

3.1.1 Introduction and Indications

Venlafaxine is a selective serotonin and norepinephrine reuptake inhibitor (SNRI) possessing much of the efficacy of tricyclic antidepressants (TCAs) without the risk of overdose and side effects associated with TCAs.

Desvenlafaxine (O-desmethylvenlafaxine), a major active metabolite of venlafaxine, appears to be a more balanced serotonin–norepinephrine drug than venlafaxine [1–3].

Structure of venlafaxine hydrochloride (Fig. 3.1) [4].
Structure of desvenlafaxine (Fig. 3.2) [5].
About venlafaxine and desvenlafaxine (Fig. 3.3)

- Venlafaxine, a selective SNRI, is a dual reuptake inhibitor that received its initial approval from the United States Food and Drug Administration in 1994. It was approved to treat depression, anxiety, and chronic pain.
- Venlafaxine possesses much of the efficacy of TCAs and is tolerated better than TCAs without the risk of overdose and myriad of side effects associated with TCAs. However, it is tolerated less well than selective serotonin reuptake inhibitors (SSRIs).

A. Fagiolini et al., *Pocket Guide to Practical Psychopharmacology*, https://doi.org/10.1007/978-3-031-80490-8_3

Fig. 3.1 Structure of
venlafaxine
hydrochloride

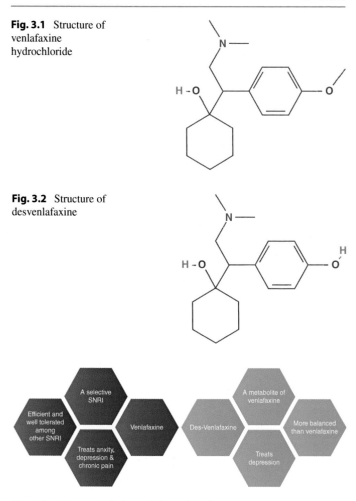

Fig. 3.2 Structure of
desvenlafaxine

Fig. 3.3 About venlafaxine and desvenlafaxine

- Desvenlafaxine is a metabolite of venlafaxine. It seems to be a
  more balanced serotonin–norepinephrine drug as compared to
  venlafaxine [2, 3, 6].
- In 2007, desvenlafaxine was approved by the United States Food
  and Drug Administration for the treatment of depression [7].

- Certain studies suggested venlafaxine to be more likely to show effects in case of remission, as compared to SSRIs. However, it is controversial based on recent meta-analyses in which venlafaxine failed to demonstrate clear merits over SSRIs [8, 1].
- Although a review study and some psychiatrists concur that venlafaxine is superior to some other antidepressants, the merits are relatively modest, which can be outweighed by the demerits, such as adverse events associated with venlafaxine [1].

What Are the Indications of Venlafaxine?

Venlafaxine is an SNRI that in the United States is indicated, in its slow-release formulation, for the treatment of adults with the following conditions: [2]

- Major depressive disorder (MDD).
- Generalized anxiety disorder (GAD).
- Social anxiety disorder (SAD).
- Panic disorder (PD).

What Are the Indications of Desvenlafaxine?

Desvenlafaxine is an SNRI indicated for treating adults with MDD [3].

3.1.2   What Are the Dosing Regimens for Venlafaxine? (Table 3.1)

Venlafaxine should be administered once daily with food. The venlafaxine capsules should be taken whole and not divided, crushed, chewed, or dissolved.

The dose of venlafaxine should be reduced gradually while discontinuing the treatment [2].

Dosing Regimen in Patients with Renal and/or Hepatic Impairment (Fig. 3.4) [2].
Dosing Regimen for Venlafaxine: Based on Indication (Fig. 3.5) [2].

Table 3.1 Dosing regimens for venlafaxine

Indication	Starting dose	Target dose	Maximum dose
Major depressive disorder (MDD)	37.5–75 mg/day	75 mg/day	225 mg/day
Generalized anxiety disorder (GAD)	37.5–75 mg/day	75 mg/day	225 mg/day
Social anxiety disorder (SAD)	75 mg/day	75 mg/day	75 mg/day
Panic disorder (PD)	37.5 mg/day	75 mg/day	225 mg/day

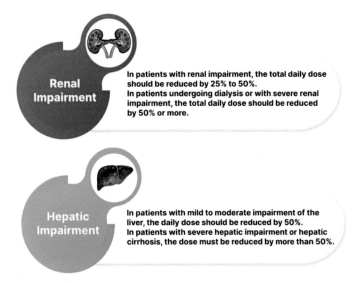

Renal Impairment

In patients with renal impairment, the total daily dose should be reduced by 25% to 50%.
In patients undergoing dialysis or with severe renal impairment, the total daily dose should be reduced by 50% or more.

Hepatic Impairment

In patients with mild to moderate impairment of the liver, the daily dose should be reduced by 50%.
In patients with severe hepatic impairment or hepatic cirrhosis, the dose must be reduced by more than 50%.

Fig. 3.4 Dosing regimen in patients with renal and/or hepatic impairment

3.1.3   What Are the Dosing Regimens for Desvenlafaxine?

The recommended dose of desvenlafaxine is 50 mg once daily with or without food. No evidence indicates that doses greater than 50 mg daily provide additional therapeutic benefits.

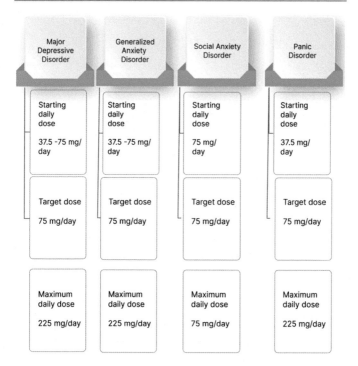

Fig. 3.5 Dosing regimen for venlafaxine

Like venlafaxine, the desvenlafaxine dose should be reduced gradually while discontinuing the treatment.

The tablets of desvenlafaxine should be taken whole without dividing, crushing, chewing, or dissolving [3].

Dosing Regimen in Patients with Renal and/or Hepatic Impairment (Fig. 3.6) [3]**.**

3.1.4   What Are the Pharmacokinetic Profiles of Venlafaxine and Desvenlafaxine?

Absorption, Distribution, Metabolism, and Excretion of Venlafaxine (Fig. 3.7) [2]**.**

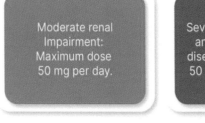

Fig. 3.6 Dosing regimen in patients with renal and/or hepatic impairment

The steady-state concentrations of venlafaxine and O-desmethylvenlafaxine are reached within 3 days of the drug intake. The time of administration (AM or PM) does not affect the pharmacokinetics of venlafaxine and O-desmethylvenlafaxine.

Absorption, Distribution, Metabolism, and Excretion of Desvenlafaxine (Fig. 3.8) [3].

The steady-state concentration of desvenlafaxine is reached within approximately 4–5 days of the drug intake (with once-daily dosing).

3.1.5 What Are the Pharmacodynamic Profiles of Venlafaxine and Desvenlafaxine?

Venlafaxine and its active metabolite desvenlafaxine are potent and selective SNRIs and weak dopamine reuptake inhibitors. Both these drugs have no significant affinity for muscarinic cholinergic,

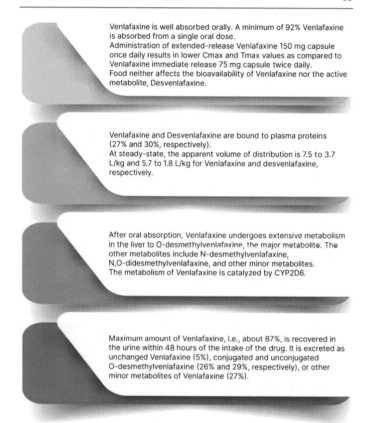

Venlafaxine is well absorbed orally. A minimum of 92% Venlafaxine is absorbed from a single oral dose.
Administration of extended-release Venlafaxine 150 mg capsule once daily results in lower Cmax and Tmax values as compared to Venlafaxine immediate release 75 mg capsule twice daily.
Food neither affects the bioavailability of Venlafaxine nor the active metabolite, Desvenlafaxine.

Venlafaxine and Desvenlafaxine are bound to plasma proteins (27% and 30%, respectively).
At steady-state, the apparent volume of distribution is 7.5 to 3.7 L/kg and 5.7 to 1.8 L/kg for Venlafaxine and desvenlafaxine, respectively.

After oral absorption, Venlafaxine undergoes extensive metabolism in the liver to O-desmethylvenlafaxine, the major metabolite. The other metabolites include N-desmethylvenlafaxine, N,O-didesmethylvenlafaxine, and other minor metabolites. The metabolism of Venlafaxine is catalyzed by CYP2D6.

Maximum amount of Venlafaxine, i.e., about 87%, is recovered in the urine within 48 hours of the intake of the drug. It is excreted as unchanged Venlafaxine (5%), conjugated and unconjugated O-desmethylvenlafaxine (26% and 29%, respectively), or other minor metabolites of Venlafaxine (27%).

Fig. 3.7 Absorption, distribution, metabolism, and excretion of venlafaxine. C_{max}: Peak plasma concentration; T_{max}: Time to reach C_{max}

α_1-adrenergic, or H_1-histaminergic receptors in vitro. These drugs also lack monoamine oxidase inhibitors (MAOI) activity [2, 3].

Electrocardiogram Changes   Venlafaxine and desvenlafaxine do not cause significant QT prolongation [2, 3].

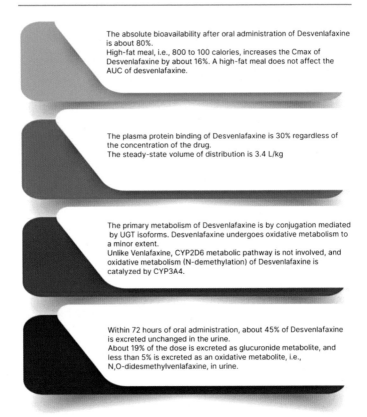

The absolute bioavailability after oral administration of Desvenlafaxine is about 80%.
High-fat meal, i.e., 800 to 100 calories, increases the Cmax of Desvenlafaxine by about 16%. A high-fat meal does not affect the AUC of desvenlafaxine.

The plasma protein binding of Desvenlafaxine is 30% regardless of the concentration of the drug.
The steady-state volume of distribution is 3.4 L/kg

The primary metabolism of Desvenlafaxine is by conjugation mediated by UGT isoforms. Desvenlafaxine undergoes oxidative metabolism to a minor extent.
Unlike Venlafaxine, CYP2D6 metabolic pathway is not involved, and oxidative metabolism (N-demethylation) of Desvenlafaxine is catalyzed by CYP3A4.

Within 72 hours of oral administration, about 45% of Desvenlafaxine is excreted unchanged in the urine.
About 19% of the dose is excreted as glucuronide metabolite, and less than 5% is excreted as an oxidative metabolite, i.e., N,O-didesmethylvenlafaxine, in urine.

Fig. 3.8 Absorption, distribution, metabolism, and excretion of desvenlafaxine

3.1.6   What Is the Mechanism of Actions of Venlafaxine and Desvenlafaxine?

Mechanism of Action of Venlafaxine.

Although the mechanism of action of this drug in treating MDD, SAD, GAD, and PD is not clear, it could be linked with norepinephrine and serotonin potentiation in the central nervous system by inhibiting their reuptake (Fig. 3.9) [2, 3].

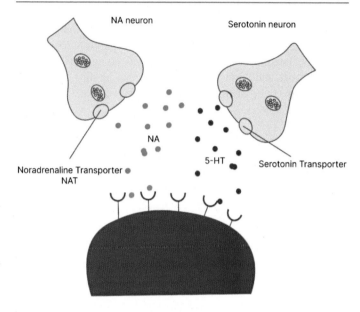

Fig. 3.9 Mechanism of action of venlafaxine

Mechanism of Action of Desvenlafaxine.

Although the exact mechanism of this drug in treating MDD is unknown, it could be linked with serotonin and norepinephrine potentiation in the central nervous system by inhibiting their reuptake. Non-clinical studies have indicated that this drug is a potent and selective SNRI [2, 3].

3.1.7 What Happens if Venlafaxine or Desvenlafaxine Is Discontinued?

Abrupt discontinuation is not recommended with venlafaxine and desvenlafaxine, as abrupt cessation of these drugs is associated with a discontinuation syndrome. Therefore, the discontinuation of these drugs should be accomplished with gradual dose tapering [2, 3].

Adverse reactions after abrupt discontinuation of serotonergic antidepressants, such as venlafaxine and desvenlafaxine, include nausea, dysphoric mood, anxiety, sweating, agitation, irritability, dizziness, headache, sensory disturbances (e.g., paresthesia—electric shock sensations), tremor, emotional lability, confusion, lethargy, insomnia, tinnitus, seizures, and hypomania [2, 3].

3.1.8 What Are the Contraindications of Venlafaxine and Desvenlafaxine?

Due to the risk of serotonin syndrome, all serotonergic medications are contraindicated with MAOIs [2, 3].

Contraindications of Venlafaxine and Desvenlafaxine (Fig. 3.10).

3.1.9 What Are the Warnings and Precautions of Venlafaxine and Desvenlafaxine?

The warnings and precautions for patients using venlafaxine and desvenlafaxine include the following (Fig. 3.11): [2, 3]

- **Increased risk of suicidal thoughts and behaviors in children, adolescents, and young adults taking antidepressants.**
  - These patients should be closely monitored for clinical worsening and the emergence of suicidal thoughts and behaviors.
  - In patients of all age groups, routine assessment for developing or worsening of suicidal thoughts and behaviors should be done.
  - Family and caretakers of the patients should observe the patients closely and communicate with the treating physicians.
  - Venlafaxine and desvenlafaxine are not approved for use in pediatric patients.

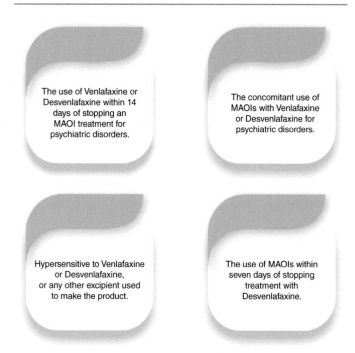

The use of Venlafaxine or Desvenlafaxine within 14 days of stopping an MAOI treatment for psychiatric disorders.

The concomitant use of MAOIs with Venlafaxine or Desvenlafaxine for psychiatric disorders.

Hypersensitive to Venlafaxine or Desvenlafaxine, or any other excipient used to make the product.

The use of MAOIs within seven days of stopping treatment with Desvenlafaxine.

Fig. 3.10 Contraindications of venlafaxine and desvenlafaxine. MAOI: Monoamine oxidase inhibitor

- **Serotonin syndrome:** Venlafaxine and desvenlafaxine increase the risk of a fatal condition called serotonin syndrome. Concomitant use of other serotonergic drugs, such as SSRIs, SNRIs, triptans, and drugs that impair the serotonin metabolism, such as MAOIs, increases the risk of serotonin syndrome. If it occurs, discontinue the use of venlafaxine and desvenlafaxine along with initiation of supportive treatment.
- **Elevated blood pressure:** Hypertension should be controlled before initiating treatment with venlafaxine or desvenlafaxine. Blood pressure should be regularly monitored during the treatment. The dose of the drug should be reduced, or the drug

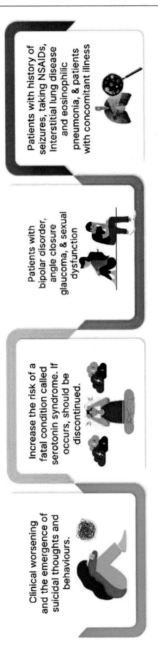

Fig. 3.11 Warnings and precautions of venlafaxine and desvenlafaxine

should be discontinued if there is a sustained increase in blood pressure.

- **Increased risk of bleeding:** Drugs interfering with serotonin reuptake inhibition, including venlafaxine and desvenlafaxine, may increase the risk of bleeding. Also, concomitant use of aspirin, nonsteroidal anti-inflammatory drugs, warfarin, other antiplatelet drugs, and other anticoagulants may also increase risk.

- **Angle-closure glaucoma:** Angle-closure glaucoma can occur in patients with untreated anatomically narrow angles if prescribed with antidepressants, including venlafaxine and desvenlafaxine.

- **Activation of mania or hypomania:** The patients should be screened for bipolar disorder. As mania was reported in MDD premarketing studies in a small proportion of patients treated with venlafaxine and desvenlafaxine, and activation of mania/ hypomania has been reported in a small percentage of patients treated with marketed antidepressant drugs, venlafaxine and desvenlafaxine should be used with caution in those with a medical or family history of mania or hypomania.

- **Discontinuation syndrome:** Venlafaxine and desvenlafaxine should not be discontinued abruptly as they may lead to symptoms, including nausea, dysphoric mood, anxiety, sweating, agitation, irritability, dizziness, headache, sensory disturbances (e.g., paresthesia—electric shock sensations), tremor, emotional lability, confusion, lethargy, insomnia, tinnitus, seizures, and hypomania. The dose should be tapered, and the patient should be monitored for discontinuation symptoms.

- **Seizures:** Cases of seizures have been observed in patients treated with venlafaxine and desvenlafaxine. Thus, these drugs should be used cautiously in patients with a seizure disorder.

- **Hyponatremia:** Can occur in association with the syndrome of inappropriate antidiuretic hormone secretion. Elderly patients may be at a greater risk of experiencing hyponatremia when treated with venlafaxine or desvenlafaxine. The treatment should be discontinued in patients with symptomatic hyponatremia, and appropriate medical management should be provided.

- **Interstitial lung disease and eosinophilic pneumonia:** These symptoms are rarely reported with venlafaxine therapy. However, these symptoms should be considered in patients on extended-release venlafaxine therapy or desvenlafaxine therapy who present with progressive dyspnea, chest discomfort, or cough. Thus, immediate medical attention should be provided to these patients, and desvenlafaxine should be discontinued.
- **Sexual dysfunction:** Venlafaxine and desvenlafaxine may cause symptoms of sexual dysfunction. In male patients, these drugs may cause decreased libido, ejaculatory delay or failure, and erectile dysfunction. In female patients, these drugs may cause delayed or absent orgasm and decreased libido.
- **Anorexia:** It may be observed in pediatric patients treated with venlafaxine extended-release medication for MDD, GAD, and SAD. The loss of weight and increased height have also been noted in premarketing studies in pediatric patients with GAD, MDD, and SAD.

3.1.10 What Are the Most Common or Most Worrisome Adverse Reactions Associated with Venlafaxine and Desvenlafaxine?

Adverse Reactions Associated with Venlafaxine.

Most common adverse reactions, i.e., incidence $\geq 5\%$ and twice that of a placebo, include nausea, constipation, dry mouth, abnormal ejaculation, sleepiness, sweating, anorexia, impotence (men), and decreased libido [2].

In addition to the adverse reactions mentioned in the below figure, appetite, height, and weight changes in pediatric patients are some other adverse reactions of venlafaxine [2].

Adverse Reactions Associated with Desvenlafaxine (Fig. 3.12).

Most common adverse reactions, i.e., incidence $\geq 5\%$ and twice that of placebo in the 50 or 100 mg dose groups, include nausea, insomnia, dizziness, hyperhidrosis, sleepiness, constipation, decreased appetite, specific male sexual function disorders, and anxiety [3].

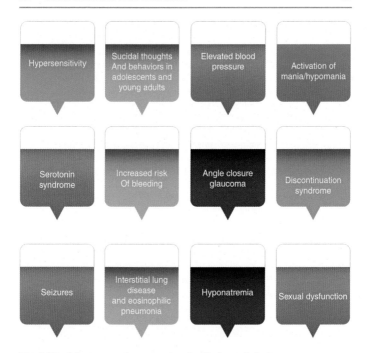

Fig. 3.12 Adverse reactions associated with desvenlafaxine

3.1.11 What Are the Clinically Important Drug Interactions Associated with Venlafaxine and Desvenlafaxine?

Clinically Important Drug Interactions Associated with Venlafaxine and Desvenlafaxine (Table 3.2).

In addition, CYP3A4 inhibitors also possess clinically important drug interactions associated with venlafaxine. Concomitant use of a CYP3A inhibitor increases the peak plasma concentrations (C_{max}) and area under the curve (AUC) of venlafaxine and the primary metabolite, desvenlafaxine. However, the interaction of CYP3A4 inhibitors with desvenlafaxine orally administered product is not clinically important, and no adjustment of dose is required [2, 3].

Table 3.2 Clinically important drug interactions associated with venlafaxine and desvenlafaxine

Monoamine oxidase inhibitors (MAOIs)	The concomitant use of venlafaxine and desvenlafaxine with MAOIs increases the risk of serotonin syndrome. Concomitant use of venlafaxine or desvenlafaxine is contraindicated with an MAOI intended to treat psychiatric disorders or within 7 days of discontinuing venlafaxine or desvenlafaxine. Venlafaxine and desvenlafaxine are contraindicated within 14 days of discontinuing an MAOI intended to treat psychiatric disorders. Concomitant use of venlafaxine or desvenlafaxine with linezolid or intravenous methylene blue is also contraindicated. Examples of MAOIs: selegiline, tranylcypromine, isocarboxazid, phenelzine, linezolid, methylene blue
Other serotonergic drugs	Concomitant use of venlafaxine and desvenlafaxine with other serotonergic drugs increases the risk or serotonin syndrome. Monitor for symptoms of serotonin syndrome and discontinue the treatment if it occurs. Examples of other serotonergic drugs: Other SNRIs, SSRIs, triptans, tricyclic antidepressants, fentanyl, lithium, tramadol, buspirone, amphetamines, tryptophan, and St. John's wort
Drugs that interfere with hemostasis	Concomitant use of venlafaxine or desvenlafaxine with an antiplatelet or anticoagulant drug may increase the risk of bleeding. It could be due to the effect on the release of serotonin by platelets. Monitor the patients for bleeding when venlafaxine or desvenlafaxine is initiated or discontinued. Examples of drugs interfering with hemostasis: Nonsteroidal anti-inflammatory drugs, warfarin, and aspirin
CYP2D6 substrates	Concomitant use of venlafaxine or desvenlafaxine increases the C_{max} and AUC of the drugs that are metabolized by CYP206, increasing the toxicity risk of the CYP2D6 substrate drug. Examples of drugs metabolized by CYP2D6: Desipramine, dextromethorphan, atomoxetine, nebivolol, perphenazine, metoprolol, and tolterodine

3.1.12 What Is the Potential for Drug Abuse When Patients Are Treated with Venlafaxine or Desvenlafaxine?

Venlafaxine and desvenlafaxine are not controlled substances.

Although venlafaxine has not been studied for its potential abuse, the clinical studies did not show any drug-seeking behavior in patients. Based on the premarketing experience, it is impossible to predict the extent of misuse, diversion, and/or abuse after the drug is in the market. Thus, the patients should be carefully monitored for signs of drug misuse or abuse [2, 3].

Is There Drug Dependence Associated with Venlafaxine or Desvenlafaxine?

Physical dependence is a state resulting from physiological adaptation due to repeated drug use, demonstrated by withdrawal signs and symptoms after sudden discontinuation or a significant reduction in the dose of a drug (Fig. 3.13) [2, 3].

3.1.13 What Happens in the Case of Venlafaxine or Desvenlafaxine Overdose?

In postmarketing experience, overdose has occurred predominantly when venlafaxine or desvenlafaxine are used in combination with alcohol and/or other drugs [2, 3].

Venlafaxine is more dangerous in overdose as compared to other SNRIs [9].

Venlafaxine or Desvenlafaxine Overdose (Fig. 3.14) [2, 3].
Management of Overdose [2, 3].

Specific antidotes for the management of venlafaxine and desvenlafaxine overdose are not available. Multiple drugs may be prescribed to manage the overdose of these antidepressant drugs. A medical toxicologist should be contacted to manage the overdose of venlafaxine or desvenlafaxine.

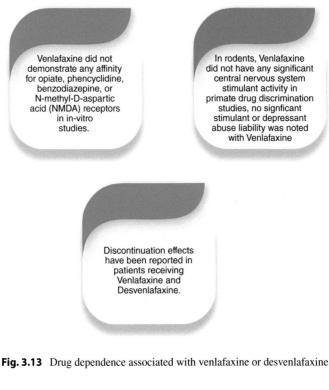

Fig. 3.13 Drug dependence associated with venlafaxine or desvenlafaxine

Fig. 3.14 Symptoms of venlafaxine or desvenlafaxine overdose

Most Commonly reported events in overdosage	Electrocardiogram changes in overdosage
• Tachycardia • Changes in level of consciousness, which could range from somnolence to coma • Mydriasis • Seizures • Vomiting	• Ventricular tachycardia • Bradycardia • Hypotension • Rhabdomyolysis • Vertigo • Liver necrosis • Serotonin syndrome • Death

3.1.14   Can Venlafaxine or Desvenlafaxine be Prescribed to Special Populations (Fig. 3.15–3.16)?

Can Venlafaxine and Desvenlafaxine Be Prescribed to Patients with Concomitant Illness?
Venlafaxine and Desvenlafaxine in Patients with Renal and Hepatic Impairment (Fig. 3.17).

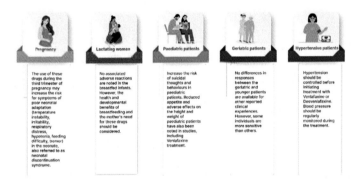

Fig. 3.15   Venlafaxine or desvenlafaxine in special populations

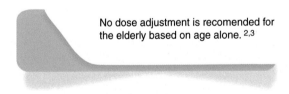

Fig. 3.16   Venlafaxine or desvenlafaxine in elderly

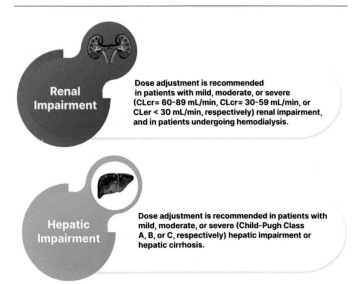

Fig. 3.17 Venlafaxine and desvenlafaxine in patients with renal and hepatic impairment. CLcr: Creatinine clearance

Fig. 3.18 Structure of duloxetine

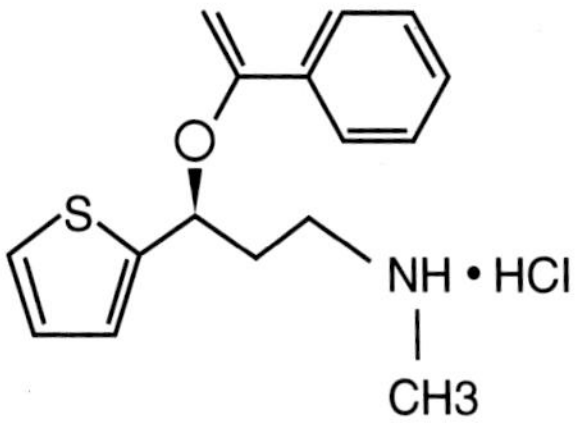

3.2   Duloxetine

3.2.1   Introduction and Indications

Duloxetine (Fig. 3.18), an SNRI introduced in 2004, has clinically significant affinity for both the serotonin and norepinephrine transporter with little affinity for other neurotransmitter receptors such as histamine or muscarinic. It is a comparatively more potent norepinephrine reuptake inhibitor (NRI) than venlafaxine.

However, it is unclear whether this increased potency translates into improved efficacy [6, 10, 11].

- Duloxetine was initially seen as an antidepressant that would be a first-line agent in depressed patients with comorbidities such as pain or stress incontinence.
- Duloxetine can be a first-line agent for patients with serious depression, including those with melancholic and psychotic subtypes [6, 10, 11].

What Are the Indications of Duloxetine (Fig. 3.19)**?**

The above indications are approved in the United States. Indications in other countries may be different.

What Are the Dosing Regimens for Duloxetine?

Duloxetine is recommended once daily, with or without food. Duloxetine delayed-release capsules should be swallowed whole. The capsule should not be crushed or chewed; it should not be opened. Missed dose of duloxetine should be taken as soon as it is remembered. Two doses of duloxetine should not be administered together [10, 11].

The Dosing Regimen for Duloxetine: Based on Indication (Fig. 3.20) [10, 11].

In countries where the 20 mg capsules are not available, starting duloxetine at 30 mg is usually beneficial.

No evidence for doses greater than 60 mg/day having additional benefit is available. However, some adverse reactions were found to be dose-dependent [10, 11].

3.2.2 What Are the Pharmacokinetic Profiles of Duloxetine?

Absorption, Distribution, Metabolism, and Excretion of Duloxetine (Fig. 3.21) [10–12].

What Is the Pharmacokinetic Profile of Duloxetine in Children and Adolescents?

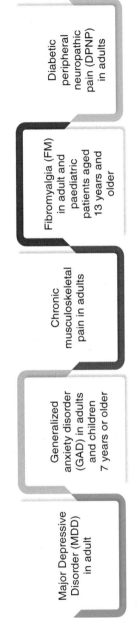

Fig. 3.19 Indications of duloxetine

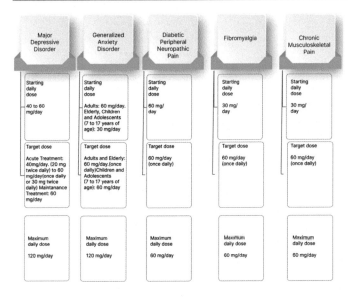

Major Depressive Disorder	Generalized Anxiety Disorder	Diabetic Peripheral Neuropathic Pain	Fibromyalgia	Chronic Musculoskeletal Pain
Starting daily dose 40 to 60 mg/day	**Starting daily dose** Adults: 60 mg/day. Elderly, Children and Adolescents (7 to 17 years of age): 30 mg/day	**Starting daily dose** 60 mg/day	**Starting daily dose** 30 mg/day	**Starting daily dose** 30 mg/day
Target dose Acute Treatment: 40mg/day. (20 mg twice daily) to 60 mg/day(once daily or 30 mg twice daily) Maintanance Treatment: 60 mg/day	**Target dose** Adults and Elderly: 60 mg/day.(once daily)Children and Adolescents (7 to 17 years of age): 60 mg/day	**Target dose** 60 mg/day (once daily)	**Target dose** 60 mg/day (once daily)	**Target dose** 60 mg/day (once daily)
Maximum daily dose 120 mg/day	**Maximum daily dose** 120 mg/day	**Maximum daily dose** 60 mg/day	**Maximum daily dose** 60 mg/day	**Maximum daily dose** 60 mg/day

Fig. 3.20 The dosing regimen for duloxetine

The steady-state plasma concentration is comparable in children between 7 and 12 years, adolescents between 13 and 17 years, and adults. However, the average steady-state concentration is about 30% lower in children and adolescents than in adults.

Duloxetine steady-state plasma concentrations in children and adolescents are mostly within the concentration range observed in adult patients [10, 11].

3.2.3 What Is the Pharmacodynamic Profile of Duloxetine?

As per preclinical studies, this drug is a potent inhibitor of neuronal norepinephrine and serotonin reuptake. It is a less potent inhibitor of dopamine reuptake.

Duloxetine has no significant affinity for histaminergic, adrenergic, cholinergic, glutamate, opioid, dopaminergic, and gamma amino butyric acid receptors in vitro. Duloxetine does not inhibit monoamine oxidase (MAO).

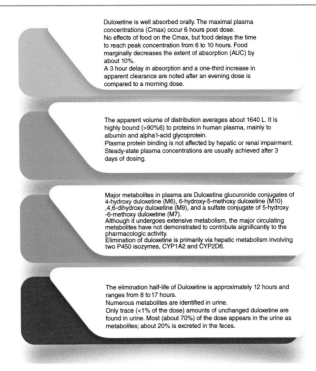

Duloxetine is well absorbed orally. The maximal plasma concentrations (Cmax) occur 6 hours post dose.
No effects of food on the Cmax, but food delays the time to reach peak concentration from 6 to 10 hours. Food marginally decreases the extent of absorption (AUC) by about 10%.
A 3 hour delay in absorption and a one-third increase in apparent clearance are noted after an evening dose is compared to a morning dose.

The apparent volume of distribution averages about 1640 L. It is highly bound (>90%6) to proteins in human plasma, mainly to albumin and alpha1-acid glycoprotein.
Plasma protein binding is not affected by hepatic or renal impairment.
Steady-state plasma concentrations are usually achieved after 3 days of dosing.

Major metabolites in plasma are Duloxetine glucuronide conjugates of 4-hydroxy duloxetine (M6), 6-hydroxy-5-methoxy duloxetine (M10) ,4,6-dihydroxy duloxetine (M9), and a sulfate conjugate of 5-hydroxy -6-methoxy duloxetine (M7).
Although it undergoes extensive metabolism, the major circulating metabolites have not demonstrated to contribute significantly to the pharmacologic activity.
Elimination of duloxetine is primarily via hepatic metabolism involving two P450 isozymes, CYP1A2 and CYP2D6.

The elimination half-life of Duloxetine is approximately 12 hours and ranges from 8 to 17 hours.
Numerous metabolites are identified in urine.
Only trace (<1% of the dose) amounts of unchanged duloxetine are found in urine. Most (about 70%) of the dose appears in the urine as metabolites; about 20% is excreted in the feces.

Fig. 3.21 Absorption, distribution, metabolism, and excretion of duloxetine

Duloxetine is in a class of medications known to affect urethral resistance; therefore, if urinary hesitation symptoms develop during treatment, it could be related to duloxetine [10, 11].

3.2.4 What Is the Mechanism of Action of Duloxetine?

The exact mechanisms of the antidepressant, anxiolytic, and central pain inhibitory actions of duloxetine in humans are unknown. However, these actions are associated with the effect to potentiate the serotonergic and noradrenergic activity in the central nervous system [10, 11].

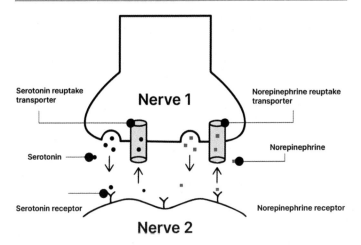

Fig. 3.22 Mechanism of action of duloxetine

Unlike the TCAs, SNRIs inhibit the reuptake of serotonin more potently than the reuptake of norepinephrine. Like most SSRIs, SNRIs have minimal or no affinity for histaminergic, muscarinic cholinergic, and adrenergic receptors.

Duloxetine also inhibits the reuptake of both serotonin and norepinephrine. Duloxetine appears to be as effective as SSRIs in treating MDD (Fig. 3.22). In more severe depression, duloxetine may have some advantages. Duloxetine does not possess significant antihistaminergic, cholinergic, and alpha1-adrenergic blocking effects [12].

3.2.5 What Happens if Duloxetine Is Discontinued (Fig. 3.23)?

Abrupt discontinuation is not recommended as it is associated with discontinuation syndrome similar to that seen with SSRI and SNRI antidepressants. Therefore, discontinuation of duloxetine should be done with a gradual tapering of the dose over at least 2 weeks to reduce the risk of discontinuation-related adverse events, also known as discontinuation syndrome.

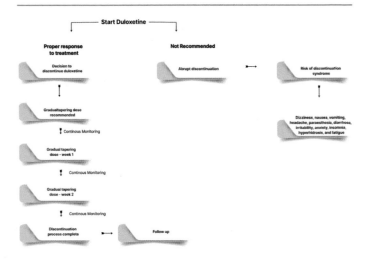

Fig. 3.23 Abrupt discontinuation of duloxetine

Adverse reactions after abrupt or tapered discontinuation of duloxetine include dizziness, nausea, vomiting, headache, paresthesia, diarrhea, irritability, anxiety, insomnia, hyperhidrosis, and fatigue [10–12].

3.2.6 What Are the Contraindications of Duloxetine?

As there is a risk of serotonin syndrome, serotonergic medications should not be taken with MAOIs. A washout is necessary when switching to MAOI, dependent on the half-life of the serotonergic agent [13].

Contraindications of Duloxetine (Fig. 3.24) [10, 11].

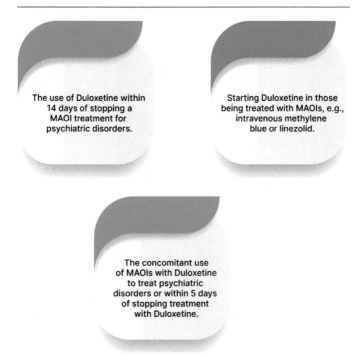

The use of Duloxetine within 14 days of stopping a MAOI treatment for psychiatric disorders.

Starting Duloxetine in those being treated with MAOIs, e.g., intravenous methylene blue or linezolid.

The concomitant use of MAOIs with Duloxetine to treat psychiatric disorders or within 5 days of stopping treatment with Duloxetine.

Fig. 3.24 Contraindications of duloxetine. MAOI: Monoamine oxidase inhibitor

3.2.7 What Are the Warnings and Precautions of Duloxetine?

- **Suicidal behaviors and thoughts in young adults and adolescents:** All patients on duloxetine treatment for depression should be monitored for worsening of symptoms and occurrence of suicidal behaviors and thoughts, particularly during the first few months of treatment and during dose modifications. Family members and caregivers should be counseled to observe for behavioral changes and to inform the doctor about any observations. The therapeutic regimen should be changed, or duloxetine should be discontinued in case of worsening depression or emergent suicidal thoughts or behaviors [10, 11].

- **Serotonin syndrome:** It occurs when duloxetine is administered alone or especially co-administered with other serotonergic agents (e.g., triptans, fentanyl, buspirone, lithium, tramadol, tricyclic antidepressants, tryptophan, St. John's Wort, and amphetamines). Duloxetine should be discontinued, and supportive treatment should be initiated when such symptoms occur. If the coadministration of duloxetine with other serotonergic drugs is clinically necessary, patients should be informed about the increased risk of serotonin syndrome, particularly during the start of treatment or when the dosage is being increased [10, 11].
- **Hepatotoxicity:** Liver failure (sometimes fatal) has been reported with duloxetine. Duloxetine should be discontinued if patient develops jaundice or other clinically significant liver issues. Duloxetine should not be resumed in these patients unless another cause can be established [10, 11].
- Duloxetine treatment is not recommended in patients with alcohol intake or evidence of chronic liver disease [10, 11].
- Dose reduction or discontinuation is recommended in case of orthostatic hypotension, falls, and syncope.
- The risk of bleeding events increases with duloxetine treatment. In addition, coadministration of duloxetine with nonsteroidal anti-inflammatory drugs, aspirin, or other drugs that affect blood coagulation may increase the risk of bleeding, and the patients should be cautioned about it.
- Duloxetine may cause severe skin reactions, including Stevens-Johnson syndrome and erythema multiforme. Duloxetine should be discontinued if symptoms, such as mucosal erosions, peeling rash, blisters, or any other sign of hypersensitivity, occur.
- Activation of mania or hypomania may be noted with duloxetine.
- Duloxetine administration in patients with untreated anatomically narrow angles may lead to angle-closure glaucoma.
- Duloxetine should be prescribed with caution in those with a history of seizure disorder.
- Blood pressure should be monitored before initiating duloxetine and periodically throughout treatment.

- Inhibitors of CYP1A2 or thioridazine should not be administered with duloxetine.
- Hyponatremia may occur in patients taking duloxetine.
- In diabetic peripheral neuropathic pain patients, minor rise in fasting blood glucose and glycosylated hemoglobin (HbA1c) may occur on duloxetine administration.
- Duloxetine should be cautiously administered in patients with conditions that slow gastric emptying.
- Urinary hesitation and retention may occur in patients taking Duloxetine [10, 11].

3.2.8 What Are the Most Common or Most Worrisome Adverse Reactions Associated with Duloxetine?

SNRIs share many of the side effects of SSRIs. For example, gastrointestinal side effects are common with SNRIs. In addition, SNRIs may have a greater propensity for causing nausea than some SSRIs.

One side effect of the SNRIs that differs from those of SSRIs is treatment-emergent hypertension. Duloxetine may also increase blood pressure; however, the rise in blood pressure is less than other SNRIs.

The more potent noradrenergic effects of duloxetine also result in various anticholinergic-like adverse effects, including dry mouth, constipation, and urinary retention. Older men might be particularly susceptible to retaining urine and should be monitored [14, 6].

Most common adverse reactions associated with duloxetine: [10, 11].

Adults Dry mouth, nausea, constipation, decreased appetite, hyperhidrosis, and somnolence.

Pediatric Patients Nausea, diarrhea, and decreased weight.

Adverse Reactions Associated with Duloxetine (Fig. 3.25) [10, 11].

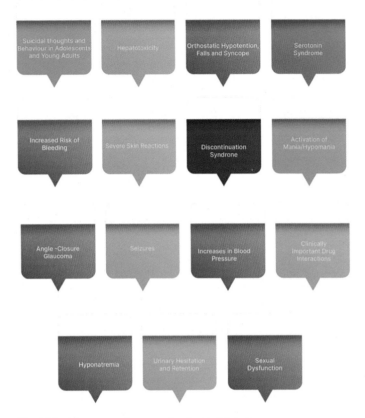

Fig. 3.25 Adverse reactions associated with duloxetine

3.2.9   What Are the Drug Interactions Associated with Duloxetine?

Duloxetine interacts with several drugs or classes of drugs and should be used with caution when used concomitantly. Warning and precautions of duloxetine should be referred to for more details on drug interactions [6, 10, 11].

Duloxetine–Drug Interactions (Fig. 3.26) [6, 10, 11].

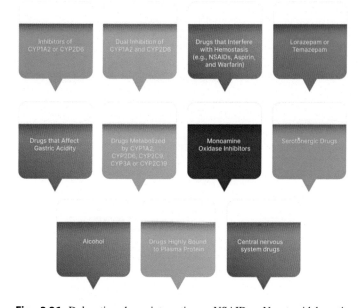

Fig. 3.26 Duloxetine–drug interactions. NSAIDs: Nonsteroidal anti-inflammatory drugs

What Are the Clinically Important Drug Interactions Associated with Duloxetine?

Duloxetine metabolism in human body is by enzymes CYP1A2 and CYP2D6 [10, 11].

Clinically Important Drug Interactions Associated with Duloxetine (Fig. 3.27) [6, 10, 11].

3.2.10 What Is the Potential for Drug Abuse When Patients Are Treated with Duloxetine?

In animal studies, no barbiturate-like (depressant) potential for abuse was noted with duloxetine. Although duloxetine has not been studied for its potential for abuse in humans, drug-seeking behavior was not noted in clinical trials.

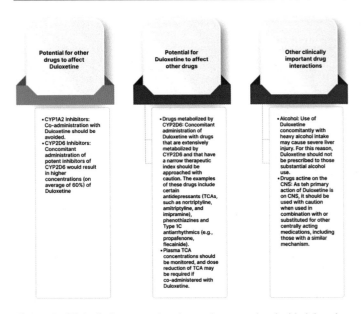

Fig. 3.27 Clinically important drug interactions associated with duloxetine. CNS: Central nervous system; CYP: Cytochrome P; TCA: Tricyclic antidepressant

Based on premarketing experience, it is impossible to predict the extent of possible misuse, diversion, or abuse of CNS active drug after it is marketed. Thus, healthcare practitioners should assess patients for drug abuse history and monitor them for any sign of abuse or misuse of duloxetine (e.g., development of tolerance, drug-seeking behavior) [10, 11].

Is Drug Dependence Associated with Duloxetine?

Duloxetine did not exhibit potential for producing dependence in rats in drug dependence studies [10, 11].

3.2.11 What Happens in the Case of Duloxetine Overdose?

Symptoms of overdose: Fatal duloxetine overdoses are more uncommon than those with venlafaxine [6].

In postmarketing experience, fatal results are reported for acute overdoses with duloxetine, primarily with mixed overdoses. The duloxetine overdoses are at doses as low as 1000 mg [10, 11].

Signs and Symptoms of Duloxetine Overdose: Alone or in Combination with Other Drugs (Fig. 3.28) [10, 11].
Management of Overdose (Fig. 3.29) [6, 10, 11].

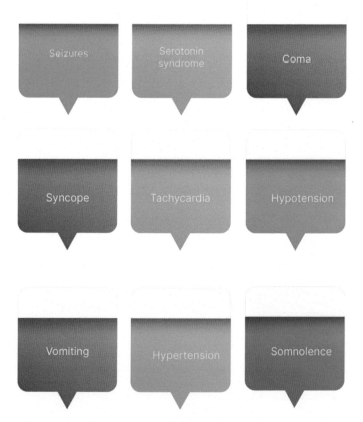

Fig. 3.28 Signs and symptoms of duloxetine overdose

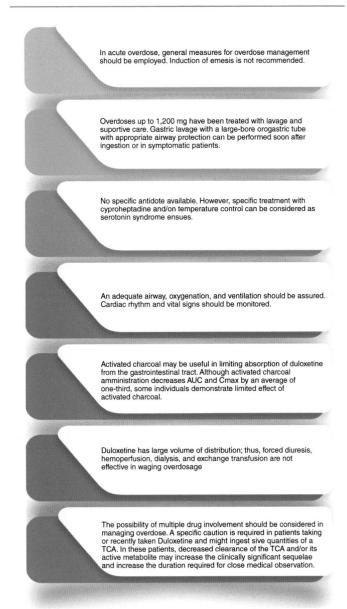

Fig. 3.29 Management of overdose. AUC: Area under the curve; C_{max}: Maximal plasma concentration; TCA: Tricyclic antidepressant

3.2.12 Can Duloxetine Be Used in Special Populations?

Can Duloxetine Be Prescribed to Pregnant Women?

Pregnancy Category C
There are no sufficient and well-controlled studies of duloxetine in pregnancy. Therefore, duloxetine should be used in pregnant women only in cases where the potential benefit justifies the potential risk [10, 11].

Can Duloxetine Be Prescribed to Lactating Mothers?

Duloxetine is present in human milk. Thus, caution should be exercised when duloxetine is administered to a nursing woman.

At steady state, the concentration of duloxetine in breast milk was about 25% that of maternal plasma, and the estimated daily infant dose was approximately 0.14% of the maternal dose [10, 11].

Can Duloxetine Be Prescribed to Pediatric Patients?

Children and adolescents treated with duloxetine should be regularly monitored for their weight and growth. The use of duloxetine in children and adolescents must balance the potential risks with the clinical requirement [10, 11].

Duloxetine in Pediatric Patients with Generalized Anxiety Disorder (GAD) and Major Depressive Disorder (MDD) (Fig. 3.30) [10, 11].

Can Duloxetine Be Prescribed to Geriatric Patients?

Based on duloxetine studies in the DPNP, GAD, MDD, FM, OA, and chronic low back pain studies, no differences in safety or effectiveness are noted between geriatric and younger patients.

Dose adjustment of duloxetine based on the patient's age is not required.

However, geriatric patients are at a higher risk of experiencing the side effect of hyponatremia when treated with SSRIs and SNRIs, including duloxetine [10, 11].

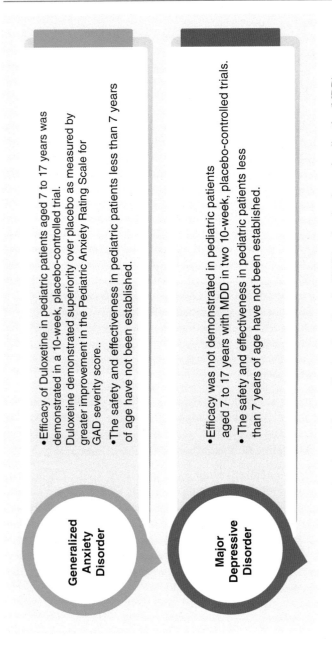

Generalized Anxiety Disorder

- Efficacy of Duloxetine in pediatric patients aged 7 to 17 years was demonstrated in a 10-week, placebo-controlled trial. Duloxetine demonstrated superiority over placebo as measured by greater improvement in the Pediatric Anxiety Rating Scale for GAD severity score..
- The safety and effectiveness in pediatric patients less than 7 years of age have not been established.

Major Depressive Disorder

- Efficacy was not demonstrated in pediatric patients aged 7 to 17 years with MDD in two 10-week, placebo-controlled trials.
- The safety and effectiveness in pediatric patients less than 7 years of age have not been established.

Fig. 3.30 Duloxetine in pediatric patients with generalized anxiety disorder (GAD) and major depressive disorder (MDD)

What Are the Effects of Gender, Race, and Smoking on Duloxetine?

Effects of Gender, Race, and Smoking Status on Duloxetine (Fig. 3.31) [10, 11].

Can Duloxetine Be Prescribed to Patients with Concomitant illness?

There is limited clinical data available to support the use of duloxetine in those with concomitant systemic illnesses [10, 11].

Duloxetine in Patients with Concomitant illness (Fig. 3.32) [10, 11].

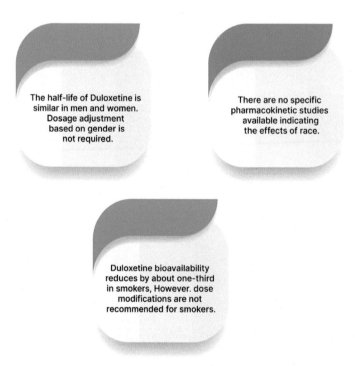

Fig. 3.31 Effects of gender, race, and smoking status on duloxetine

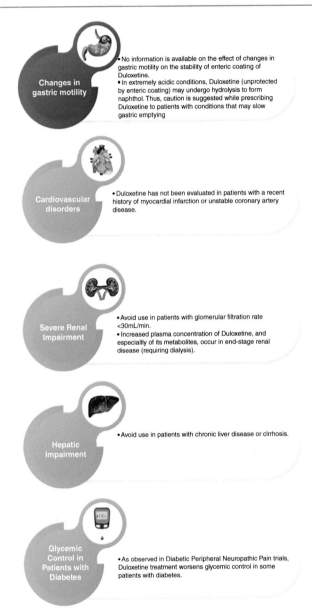

Fig. 3.32 Duloxetine in patients with concomitant illness

References

1. Liebowitz MR, Tourian KA. Efficacy safety and tolerability of Desvenlafaxine 50 mg/d for the treatment of major depressive disorder. Prim Care Companion J Clin Psychiatry. 2010; https://doi.org/10.4088/PCC.09r00845blu.

2. The United States Food and Drug Administration. Highlights of prescribing information. EFFEXOR XR® (venlafaxine extended-release) capsules. Updated 08/2023. Available from: https://www.accessdata.fda.gov/drugsatfda_docs/label/2023/020699s118lbl.pdf.

3. The United States Food and Drug Administration. Highlights of prescribing information. DESVENLAFAXINE extended-release tablets. Updated 08/2023. Available from: https://www.accessdata.fda.gov/drugsatfda_docs/label/2023/021992s051lbl.pdf.

4. National Library of Medicine. Venlafaxine. Available from: https://pubchem.ncbi.nlm.nih.gov/compound/Venlafaxine. Accessed on Jan 18, 2023.

5. National Library of Medicine. Desvenlafaxine. Available from: https://pubchem.ncbi.nlm.nih.gov/compound/Desvenlafaxine#section=2D-Structure. Accessed on Jan 18, 2023.

6. Taylor DM, Barnes TRE, Young AH. Chapter 3: Depression and anxiety disorders. In: The Maudsley® prescribing guidelines in psychiatry. 14th ed. Wiley; 2021.

7. Reddy S, Kane C, Pitrosky B, Musgnung J, Ninan PT, Guico-Pabia CJ. Clinical utility of desvenlafaxine 50 mg/d for treating MDD: a review of two randomized placebo-controlled trials for the practicing physician. Curr Med Res Opin. 2010;26(1):139–50. https://doi.org/10.1185/03007990903408678.

8. Weinmann S, Becker T, Koesters M. Re-evaluation of the efficacy and tolerability of venlafaxine vs SSRI: meta-analysis. Psychopharmacology. 2008;196(4):511–20. https://doi.org/10.1007/s00213-007-0975-9.

9. Taylor D, Lenox-Smith A, Bradley A. A review of the suitability of duloxetine and venlafaxine for use in patients with depression in primary care with a focus on cardiovascular safety suicide and mortality due to antidepressant overdose. Ther Adv Psychopharmacol. 2013;3(3):151–61. https://doi.org/10.1177/2045125312472890.

10. The United States Food and Drug Administration. Highlights of prescribing information. Cymbalta™ (Duloxetine Delayed-Release Capsules) for Oral Use. Updated 08/2023. Available from: https://pi.lilly.com/us/cymbalta-pi.pdf.

11. Summary of Product Characteristics. Cymbalta 30mg hard gastro-resistant capsules. Updated June 11, 2020. Available from: https://www.medicines.org.uk/emc/product/3880/smpc.

12. The United States Food and Drug Administration. Highlights of prescribing information. Drizalma Sprinkle™ (duloxetine delayed-release capsules). Updated 04/2020. Available from: https://www.accessdata.fda.gov/drugsatfda_docs/label/2021/212516s002lbl.pdf.
13. Edinoff AN, Swinford CR, Odisho AS, Burroughs CR, Stark CW, Raslan WA, Cornett EM, Kaye AM, Kaye AD. Clinically relevant drug interactions with monoamine oxidase inhibitors. Health Psychol Res. 2022;10(4):10.52965/001c.39576.
14. Whiskey E, Taylor D. A review of the adverse effects and safety of noradrenergic antidepressants. J Psychopharmacol. 2013;27(8):732–9. https://doi.org/10.1177/0269881113492027.